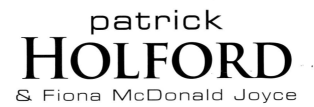

patrick
HOLFORD
& Fiona McDonald Joyce

THE
10 SECRETS
OF 100% HEALTH
COOKBOOK

SIMPLE AND DELICIOUS
RECIPES FOR OPTIMUM HEALTH

piatkus

Essex County Council

30130203229009

PIATKUS

First published in Great Britain in 2012 by Piatkus
Copyright © Patrick Holford and Fiona McDonald Joyce 2012
The moral right of the authors has been asserted.

All rights reserved.
No part of this publication may be reproduced, stored in a retrieval system, or transmitted in any form or by any means, without the prior permission in writing of the publisher, nor be otherwise circulated in any form of binding or cover other than that in which it is published and without a similar condition including this condition being imposed on the subsequent purchaser.

A CIP catalogue record for this book is available from the British Library.

ISBN 978-0-7499-5677-6

Printed and bound in China by C&C Offset Printing Co., Ltd.
Design: Emil Dacanay at D.R. ink
Recipe photography: Ian Greig Garlick
Home economist: Lorna Brash

Piatkus
An imprint of
Little, Brown Book Group
100 Victoria Embankment
London EC4Y 0DY

An Hachette UK Company
www.hachette.co.uk

www.piatkus.co.uk

Picture credits:
pp.17 © Vitalina Rybakova/istockphoto, pp.23 © Clint Scholz/istockphoto, pp.42 © Olga Lyubkina/istockphoto, pp.69 © Василий Тороус/istockphoto, pp.74 © susandaniels/istockphoto.

All other photos © Ian Greig Garlick.

With this book you are entitled to A FREE ONLINE HEALTH CHECK.
Go to www.patrickholford.com to get your free health check today.
Plus £5 OFF YOUR 100% HEALTH PROGRAMME (special price £19.95).
To obtain your discount use the following special code: 10SECUK488

About the authors

Patrick Holford, BSc, DipION, FBANT, NTCRP is a leading pioneer in new approaches to health and nutrition. He is the author of over 30 health books, translated into over 20 languages and selling over a million copies worldwide. In 1984 he founded the Institute for Optimum Nutrition, an independent educational charity and leading training institute for nutritional therapists. He is chief executive of the Food for the Brain Foundation and director of the Brain Bio Centre, the foundation's treatment centre. He is an honorary fellow of the British Association for Applied Nutrition and Nutritional Therapy, as well as a member of the Nutrition Therapy Council.

Fiona McDonald Joyce, DipION is a nutritional therapist and cookery consultant who specialises in creating healthy recipes that don't compromise on taste. With Patrick, Fiona is the co-author of *The Low-GL Diet Cookbook, Smart Food for Smart Kids, The 9-day Liver Detox, Food GLorious Food* and *The Perfect Pregnancy Plan*.

Acknowledgments

Patrick I would like to thank Jo, my wonderful assistant, and my wife Gaby, who not only takes good care of me as I write from dawn to dusk, but also tries and tests all sorts of culinary ideas. Also, I'd like to thank my daughter Jade and step-daughter Lola, who try out the recipes and let us know when something needs a tweak. Between them I am well fed.

Fiona I would like to thank my husband Nick for his usual patience and practical help and my new kitchen helper, two-year-old Oliver. I'm also grateful to Gill, Jillian and Zoe, for their help and support in producing another beautiful book. I would also like to thank Jessica Wilson for her painstaking work providing the scoring for the recipes.

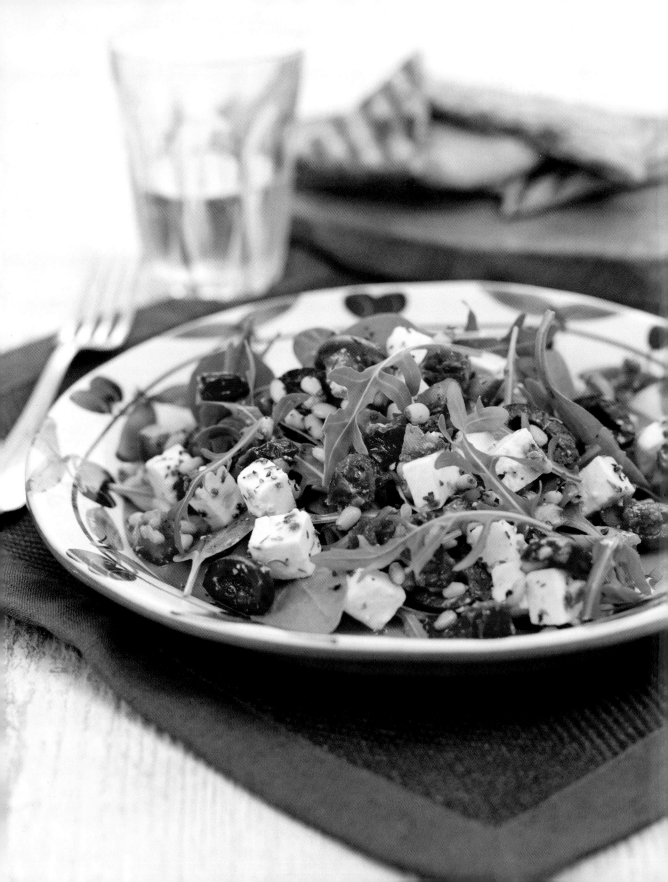

Contents

Introduction

It's hardly surprising that many people who follow popular advice on healthy eating become confused, because there are so many contradictions. One week we're told that antioxidants are essential for good health, the next week they are declared unimportant (and what are they anyway you may ask!). Fats should be avoided, so we are told. Then, it's not fat but carbohydrates that are bad news. We believe that milk is an essential staple food, but then we find out that its consumption is linked to cancer. What on earth should we be eating to stay healthy?

This is a question I've been exploring for over 30 years, by keeping up with thousands of scientific studies and by studying our body's natural design and our evolving diet and its effects on our health. One thing is clear to me: the foods that most of us are eating in our modern world are *not* the key to staying healthy. Despite living longer, which is largely ascribed to not dying young – for example, from infectious diseases – we actually have fewer *healthy* years and more years of decrepitude, suffering from the largely modern diseases of obesity, diabetes, heart disease, cancer, arthritis and Alzheimer's disease.

In 2000 I realised that perhaps the best way to find out what kind of diet would keep people 100 per cent healthy would be to ask those people who are already enjoying 100 per cent health, or who are close to it, what foods they regularly eat. To this end, I created a questionnaire – the 100% Health Check.

By 2010, almost 60,000 people had completed it. They discovered that their health could range from 'in the red', with a health score of less than 40 per cent, to 'in the green' with a health score of over 80 per cent. My team and I then analysed the results, looking particularly at the question of which foods and food groups predicted not only overall health but also immunity, digestive, hormonal and mental health, energy level and food intolerances. The results, summarised in the next chapter, were not only statistically significant at the highest level, but remarkably consistent with what is unfolding in the world of nutritional science and our understanding of humanity's evolutionary diet.

The research question we set out to ask was, *which foods increase or decrease a person's chances of being 'in the green' or 'in the red', and how much of any food is optimal?*

The results were fascinating. Take sugar consumption as an example. The results showed that your chances of being in poor health more than double if you eat three or more sugary snacks per day. Sceptics would rightly say that this strong 'association' – in this case between sugar and poor health – doesn't prove 'cause'. (For example, perhaps people who eat more sugar also smoke more and the sugar–health association is just coincidental. These are the kinds of confounding factors we control for in the analysis and, in this case, the pattern holds true for non-smokers as well as smokers). But, in fact, there is now more than enough evidence that high sugar consumption does cause ill health, including weight gain, diabetes, cardiovascular disease and cancer. This association is not surprising when you consider the diet we were designed to eat, known as our 'evolutionary diet'. The average hunter-gatherer would have consumed close to no sugar but in the Western world we now consume, on average, over 50kg (over 100lb) of sugar a year.

In my book *The 10 Secrets of 100% Healthy People* I examine the evidence to give you the ten golden rules that are consistent with the diet and lifestyle of the most healthy people, those who scored closest to 100 per cent. The purpose of this book is to turn what I outlined about diet in that book – and in *The 10 Secrets of Healthy Ageing* – into delicious and delightful recipes, menus and health habits. A saying often attributed to Mark Twain is, 'Everybody talks about the weather but nobody does anything about it.' This book is about 'doing' what's necessary to help you keep your diet healthy in a way that is highly enjoyable. It is also about hard-wiring those healthy principles by generating a new set of eating habits. However, it's not some kind of austere discipline, because what will make it succeed for you is how good you will feel afterwards.

To this end I enrolled Fiona McDonald Joyce, our kitchen wizard, who is a great cook as well as being a nutritional therapist and a mother. Her tasty recipes have tempted many people to eat healthily, and her books *Food GLorious Food*, *The Low-GL Diet Cookbook* and *Smart Food for Smart Kids*, have been enjoyed by thousands.

Together we have created a simple set of daily targets, recipes and menus to help you to acquire new habits that will increase your health as well as preventing a plethora of diseases in the future.

Learn more about yourself by discovering your health score

If you would like to discover your health score, you can complete the 100% Health Check online (you can find it on my website www.patrickholford.com). It has 229 questions and takes about 20 minutes. It is free to complete and gives you your health score, with 100 per cent being optimal health. The survey also identifies those health areas that are your weakest and that warrant attention. For a small fee you can also receive an in-depth analysis and a personal health programme to help you increase your level of health to move closer to 100 per cent. Thousands of people have taken this option and have seen their health improve, often to levels previously not experienced. I receive letters and emails every month from people expressing their gratitude for learning how to transform their health. Eamon, for example, lost 44.5kg (100lb) in weight; Karen once suffered with digestive problems but these have now disappeared, and instead of waking up lacking in energy she now starts each day fully alert; for Elaine, her devastating PMS is now a thing of the past. (As a reader of this book, you are entitled to a £5 discount on your full 100% Health Programme – see page 2.)

Hard-wiring healthy habits

It takes roughly three weeks to break a habit, six weeks to make a new habit and 36 weeks (eight months) to hard-wire a habit. In this book you'll find a simple way to achieve your daily target of health essentials.

It includes daily menu options for one week, which you can chop and change, giving you an achievable way to generate your new healthy-eating habits. This will give you a workable way to enhance your health and stay free from disease, while enjoying delicious food, recipes and daily menus. And you'll enjoy some good side effects: you'll have more energy for exercise and for resolving the stresses of daily life, which are also an essential part of being 100 per cent healthy. But the cornerstone for establishing a truly healthy lifestyle starts with taking charge of the one thing you have control over – that is, what you put in your mouth.

About this book

PART ONE explains the secrets of 100 per cent healthy people: how to eat digestion-friendly foods, all about the anti-ageing antioxidants, meals that burn fat, and the essential fats that boost your mood. I cover the six dietary secrets explained in *The 10 Secrets of 100% Healthy People* and follow these with sections on how our mental attitude affects the way we eat. Within each of the ten sections in Chapter 2 you will find some simple guidelines for you to follow to increase your level of health, and I will explain how these are incorporated into the recipes and menus. This will enable you to follow the principles 'freestyle' or just select the correct combination of recipes to achieve your goals – or you may choose to follow the daily menus, where all the work is done for you. Fiona and I recommend you follow at least four days of daily menus to get the hang of the diet before going 'freestyle'.

PART TWO gives you over 75 tried-and-tested recipes that comply with the guidelines set out in Part One, as well as advice on everything from the healthiest cooking methods, types of salt and cooking oils to use and even the best – and worst – pans. In addition to a week's menu plans, there is a table of all the recipes to provide an easy reference guide when planning your meals. The table provides scores for essential elements of this healthy diet, so that you can, for example, choose the combination of meals that will give you a good balance of particular nutrients over a day and help you to stay in good shape if you are a healthy weight or to lose pounds if you are too heavy.

Each recipe also contains Cook's Notes, which show its suitability for special diets as well as covering practical issues such as being able to be cooked in advance or frozen. In short, Part Two aims to be eminently practical, making it as easy as possible to change your dietary habits and follow my advice – even for novice cooks or complete beginners.

Wishing you the very best of health,

Patrick Holford

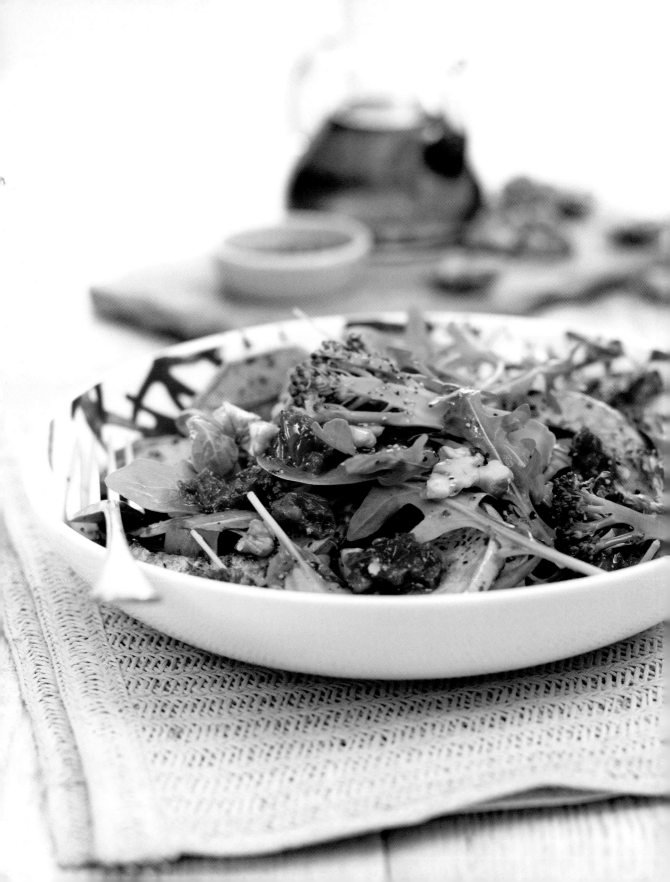

PART ONE

DEFINING 100% HEALTH AND THE PERFECT DIET

By Patrick Holford

Chapter 1 Are You 100 Per Cent Healthy?

IMAGINE THE FAIRY GODMOTHER of health had waved her magic wand and you were now 100 per cent healthy. How would you know? How would you feel? One person described their new-found health as 'being blissfully unaware of my body – no aches, pains, indigestion or tiredness. Nothing wrong!' Others describe it as having no headaches, bloating, indigestion, dry skin, colds or infections. That's certainly a large part of it. But health isn't just an absence of illness, it's also a positive state – an abundance of vitality or well-being. Apart from a lack of aches and pains, the following are the most commonly reported benefits people following my 100 per cent health principles report:

- Waking up alert
- Having loads of energy
- A sharp mind
- A balanced mood
- Good motivation
- Skin that looks good
- Effortless weight loss (if overweight)

The habits of 100 per cent healthy people

We often hear how certain diet or lifestyle habits will increase our chances of suffering from disease, the assumption being that if we don't do these things – for example, smoking or eating junk food – we won't get sick. But how can we improve our chances of good health? Our 100% Health Survey has enabled my team and I to look at the other side of the coin and discover what it is that healthy people do that unhealthy people don't.

We've used this method of analysis, for example, to investigate what a perfect diet is likely to be. To do this we took the healthiest people – those in 'optimum health' who scored above 81 per cent – and compared them with the unhealthiest people – those in 'poor or very poor health' who scored below 60 per cent – to see if there were any significant differences in their dietary habits.

Bad-news foods

The results highlighted some very interesting differences in diet. One of the most striking comparisons – and most pertinent, given the rise in cases of obesity and diabetes – was that for sugar intake, which I touched upon in the Introduction.

If you look at the chart below, you'll see on the left that your chance of being in optimal health increases six-fold, from 2 per cent to 12 per cent, if you have no sugary snacks in a day versus three or more. Conversely, on the right, your chance of being in poor health more than doubles if you have three or more sugary snacks. You'll also notice that the more you have the worse off you are.

So sugary snacks can be considered 'bad-news foods' because they have a detrimental effect on our health, but what other foods did we find that were associated with worsening your health?

The impact of sugary foods on your chances of being in poor or optimal health

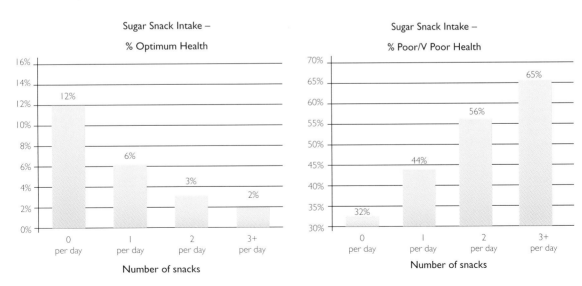

A similar, consistent pattern was seen for salt, refined food, caffeinated drinks (tea, coffee and cola), followed by wheat and dairy products (milk and cheese) and red meat. Despite being staple foods in the Western diet, the higher a person's consumption of wheat or milk products the greater were their chances of being in poor health.

Good-news foods

Exactly the opposite pattern was seen for fruit and vegetables, nuts and seeds, oily fish and drinking sufficient water. And although our results endorse the government's 'five a day' campaign, it found that the healthiest people were eating eight or more servings of fruit and vegetables. A person eating three or more pieces of fruit a day was almost twice as likely to be in optimal health as a person eating none. Fresh fruit and vegetables, together with herbs and spices, are the best sources of anti-ageing antioxidants. Ensuring you have a high daily intake of antioxidants is one of the secrets of 100 per cent healthy people. How to do this is explained on page 35 – and of course such ingredients are major constituents of the recipes.

We also found that eating only one serving a week of oily fish didn't appear to make any difference to health ratings, compared to those who ate none. But eating three or more servings of oily fish almost doubled a person's chances of being in optimal health. For this reason you'll find a lot of fish-based recipes, and recipes using vegetarian sources of omega-3 fats, particularly chia, flax and pumpkin seeds, in your daily menus. Taking in enough omega-3 fats on a daily basis is an essential habit of 100 per cent healthy people, as you'll see on page 39.

One of the single best predictors of health was a person's water consumption. Keeping yourself well hydrated, as you'll see in Chapter 2, is one of the secrets of 100 per cent healthy people. In the survey, those who drank the equivalent of eight or more glasses of water a day were twice as likely to be in optimal health.

The chart opposite summarises the results of our survey.

Good and bad foods in relation to key health factors

	Overall Health	Energy/ blood sugar	Digestion	Food sensitivity	Immunity	Hormones (male)	Hormones (female)	Mind & mood
Sugary snacks	XXX	XXX	XXX	XXX	XXX	XX	XXX	XXX
Salt	XXX	XXX	XX	XXX	XX	XXX	XXX	XXX
Refined foods	XXX	XXX	XX	XXX	XX	XX	XXX	XX
Tea/coffee	XXX	XXX	XX	XXX	XX	XXX	XX	XX
Wheat	XXX	XXX	XX	XXX	XX	XX	XX	XX
Sugar	XXX	XXX	XX	XX	XX	XXX	XX	XX
Processed foods	XXX	XXX	XX	XX	XX	XX	XXX	XX
Dairy	XXX	XXX	XX	XXX	XX	X	XX	XX
Red meat	XX	X	X	X	XX	XX		XX
Alcohol	X	X	X	X	X		XX	
Water	✓✓	✓✓✓	✓	✓✓	✓	✓	✓✓	✓
Oily fish	✓✓	✓✓	✓	✓✓	✓	✓✓	✓	✓✓
Fresh veg	✓✓	✓✓✓	✓✓	✓✓✓	✓✓	✓✓	✓✓✓	✓✓
Fresh fruit	✓✓✓	✓✓✓	✓✓	✓✓✓	✓✓	✓✓	✓✓✓	✓✓
Nuts/seeds	✓✓✓	✓✓✓	✓✓	✓✓✓	✓✓	✓✓✓	✓✓	✓✓✓

Key: This chart shows the apparent impact of increasing consumption of each food for key health factors
X = Moderate negative impact   XX= strong negative impact   XXX= very strong negative impact
✓ = Moderate positive impact   ✓✓= strong positive impact   ✓✓✓= very strong positive impact

We were also able to look more closely at the foods that are associated with various aspects of health, such as a person's energy and stress levels, hormonal balance, mental health, digestive health, immunity and skin condition. As you can see in the chart above, a consistent pattern of good and bad foods emerges. The more fruit, vegetables, oily fish, seeds, nuts and water you consume the greater are your chances of being in optimal health, while the more sugary foods, caffeinated drinks, red meat, wheat, dairy products, refined food and salt you consume the fewer are your chances.

Eating for optimal health

If the lifestyles of these healthy people explain their good health and well-being, then following these simple recommendations can be a blueprint for achieving optimal health:

1. Reduce wheat consumption to a maximum of one serving per day (of bread, pasta, pizza and so on).
2. Eliminate sugar-based snacks or limit these products to very occasional use.
3. Avoid adding salt to food, eliminate or minimise the consumption of salted snacks and reduce your use of salted, processed food.
4. Reduce your intake of dairy products to a maximum of one serving per day.
5. Reduce consumption of refined foods (that is, white bread, flour, rice and so on) to a maximum of one serving a day.
6. Increase consumption of fresh fruit and vegetables to a combined total of eight to ten servings a day.
7. Eliminate tea/coffee consumption, or limit these to very occasional use.
8. Reduce the consumption of red meat to a maximum of two servings per week, or three if one is a naturally lean game meat such as venison.
9. Increase consumption of oily fish to three servings per week.
10. Increase the consumption of fresh, raw seeds and nuts to three servings per day.
11. Increase your intake of water to eight glasses per day.

These are not only the secrets of optimal health, they are also the secrets for living a long and healthy life. In my book *The 10 Secrets of 100% Healthy Ageing*, it is following these principles that gives you the best odds for adding years to your life – and life to your years.

A diet from the past

The recommendations given above are very consistent with the kinds of foods we would have eaten thousands of years ago, when hunter-gatherers ate no dairy products and very little gluten-containing grains (such as wheat). In fact, the increase in consumption of carbohydrates, often in the form of cereals, bread and pasta, as well as sweet foods, is the most likely reason for the continuing epidemic of obesity, as well as many other chronic diseases. As you'll see in Chapter 2, what is called a low-GL (glycemic load) diet – with fewer grains and relatively more protein either from fish or beans, nuts and seeds – is consistent with promoting rapid weight loss and recovery of blood sugar balance, which is lost when too many carbohydrates are routinely eaten.

The increased consumption of meat and dairy products is one of the most likely reasons for the epidemic in breast and prostate cancers, the incidences of which are incredibly low in cultures whose diets excludes these foods, together with those that are high GL.

There is also growing evidence that avoiding eating fat is wrong. Not only is our ever-increasing epidemic of depression and aggression linked to a lack of omega-3 fats (found in oily fish) but also eating those foods may well be essential to the development of both our body and mind. One theory about the cause of the leap in intelligence of *Homo sapiens* was that it was probably driven by eating a high intake of seafood, found in wetlands, swamp lands and along the water's edge, providing the essential fats for the evolution of a smarter brain.

A lack of omega-3 fats is also strongly linked to heart disease and inflammatory diseases such as arthritis, which are, once again, endemic in the Western world. So too is a lack of vitamin D, which is made in the skin in the presence of sunlight. The best dietary source of vitamin D is oily fish, followed by eggs, both of which become essential for people living in northern Europe, especially during the winter months when there simply isn't enough intensity of strong sunlight. In Chapter 2, section 5, I give you the low down on what you need and how to get it from food.

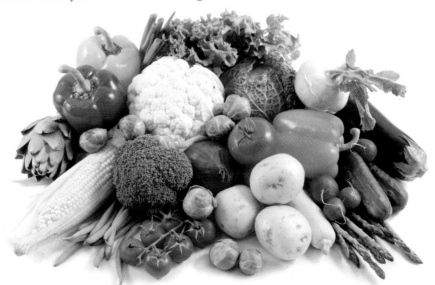

The homocysteine factor

Many of the foods that are beneficial to us – usually whole foods – are naturally rich in vital B vitamins. Vitamin B_{12} is found only in animal-based foods, and is abundant in fish. These nutrients, together with zinc (found in seeds and nuts) and tri-methyl-glycine (TMG – found in eggs and root vegetables) are vital for another key attribute of 100 per cent healthy people – that is a low homocysteine level.

Homocysteine is a type of protein produced by the body and found in the blood. Of all the biological markers of health, your blood plasma level of homocysteine is the most predictive of overall health and of risk of death from all causes. Homocysteine should be present in very low quantities – the lower your level the longer you will live and the less are your chances of suffering from cardiovascular disease, stroke, cancer, osteoporosis and Alzheimer's disease. To find your homocysteine level you will need to have it checked by a blood test. You want to have a level below 7 mmol/l for optimal health. You can organise a blood test either from your GP or you can purchase a home test kit (see Resources).

The reason why your homocysteine level is so predictive is that it reflects a vital process in your body called 'methylation'. This is one of the main ways the body keeps itself in chemical balance, finely adjusting the levels of all sorts of essential biochemicals, from adrenalin to insulin. Getting enough B vitamins from whole foods is the fuel that allows these transforming processes to run smoothly, making you feel better. A low homocysteine level is associated with better energy, mood and memory. For this reason our recipes are packed with ingredients rich in B vitamins. Chapter 2, section 3 explains homocysteine in more detail.

Defining optimum living

There's more to health than just diet and so, although this is a cookbook, we want you to be aware of the other elements to consider alongside the healthy diet we are promoting here. We contacted the top 200 healthiest people from our survey (they had all scored in the optimum range), to ask them to what they attributed their high health scores. Of the 200, 101 completed our survey and confirmed that they were still healthy. The factors they considered extremely important for health were, in order of importance: state of mind (85 per cent), nutrition (84 per cent), exercise (63 per cent), relationships (58 per cent), spirituality (44 per cent) and heredity or luck (9 per cent). Many of these factors have a relationship to the foods we eat:

Exercise Ninety-two per cent of the healthiest people considered themselves to be moderately fit, most doing three or more hours of exercise a week. Half did some form of vital-energy-generating exercise, such as t'ai chi, qigong (chi gung), yoga, Psychocalisthenics or meditation. Increasing your 'chi', or vital energy, is fundamental to Chinese medicine and certain foods provide the most vitality. I'll be explaining about these and the types of foods you need to eat to optimise fitness. The older you are the more protein you will need to help maintain muscle mass, although this is not a substitute for exercising, just a prerequisite.

Relationships Eighty per cent were in a couple and 85 per cent rated their primary relationship as good or excellent. Having a good relationship with food is also essential for health, as I will explain in Chapter 2, section 9.

Closeness to nature Ninety-three per cent considered spending time in nature and natural environments to be important to their state of mind. The food you choose to eat and your relationship to the environment is a subject we'll be exploring as another piece of the 100 per cent health equation.

Spirituality and direction in life Among the healthiest people, 83 per cent believed in God, a higher power or consciousness, and 81 per cent considered themselves spiritual. Sixty-one per cent described themselves as fulfilled, whereas 73 per cent described themselves as happy, and 78 per cent had a clear sense of purpose or direction in life.

Food is life. Our bodies are made from it, and food nourishes the body and the soul. Connecting with the food you eat – growing it, choosing local produce, eating in season, preparing and enjoying it with gratitude, or saying grace, if you are that way inclined – are all part of a healthy relationship with food. Eating consciously, including chewing your food, all makes a difference to how you feel. We'll be exploring this in more detail later.

The fact that this group of very healthy people have a number of shared habits, attitudes and attributes doesn't prove that these cause good health as such, but it's interesting to see what healthy people do and what they consider to be the secret of their good health. It certainly suggests that you have the power to transform your health by changing your diet, your lifestyle and your attitude towards life and the food you eat. These are the secrets of 100 per cent healthy living.

Chapter 2 The Dietary Secrets of 100% Health

THERE ARE TEN ASPECTS to enjoying food for the best of health, ranging from the groups of foods that support the essential processes necessary to ensure your body and brain work efficiently (based on the six dietary secrets explained in *The 10 Secrets of 100% Healthy People*) to the way you eat and prepare food, and the attitude you have towards it. In this chapter I provide you with the background to each aspect, to explain the rationale behind the recipes and menu plans we have devised for you in Part Two.

1: Choose digestion-friendly foods

Having a well-functioning and healthy digestive system is essential for good health, because every molecule in your body comes from what you put into your mouth, and your digestion needs to be in good working order so that your body can absorb the nutrients from the foods you eat. So, what is it you need to eat to benefit from healthy digestion? Most people would immediately say 'high-fibre foods', and this is partly true, but not all dietary fibres are the same.

The biggest changes in the modern-day diet, compared to that of our hunter-gatherer ancestors, is a massive increase in the intake of wheat, milk, sugar and refined foods and a corresponding decrease in fruit, vegetables, nuts and seeds. This not only equates to a massive reduction in dietary fibre, from an average of over 35g (1¼oz) a day to today's average of less than 10g (¼oz), but there is also a reason why a diet high in wheat, dairy and sugar is bad news for your digestive system.

Our deadly bread

The modern love affair with wheat stems from the fact that it is high in glutenous proteins, predominantly gliadin, which forms bubbles when you bake it with sugar-activated yeast (sugar is added to make a 'lighter' loaf). Gliadin is also somewhat addictive, making opioid-like proteins called gliadorphins.

Gliadin is a digestive irritant and many people develop some degree of intolerance or allergy to wheat. There is no gliadin in oats, and much less in rye or barley, making these grains much more digestion friendly. Both barley and oats contain soluble fibres, which means that their fibres absorb more water, increasing the bulk of digested food passing through the gut. You benefit from this by having regular bowel movements. Wheat fibre is insoluble, however, and hence absorbs little water.

You can see this by simply dropping a heaped teaspoon of oat bran into one glass of water and then doing the same with another glass using wheat bran. You'll see that the oat bran absorbs several times its own volume in water whereas wheat bran changes very little. So, eating less wheat but more oats is good for your digestion.

Avoiding common food allergens

Although gliadin isn't great news for any of us, for people with a severe allergy, called coeliac disease, it can literally be deadly as it can cause severe damage to the digestive tract, to the extent that the sufferer is unable to absorb essential nutrients from foods. About one in a hundred people has coeliac disease, which is often undiagnosed, but many more have an intolerance to wheat. The leading charity, Allergy UK, estimates that up to 45 per cent of the UK population suffers from some degree of food intolerance.

The most common allergenic foods are milk, wheat or gliadin and yeast. Although dairy products have become a staple food, consuming them in adulthood is not part of our evolutionary design – no animals continue to consume milk beyond infancy. Many people, perhaps one in four, produce antibodies against milk proteins, which activate the immune system and promote inflammation. Countries that consume the most dairy products also have the highest rates of breast and prostate cancer. This is almost certainly because milk naturally contains cell growth promoters, which are designed for babies, not for adults.

Therefore, it is generally advisable to minimise dairy products, by not consuming them every day. If you suspect you might be allergic to dairy products, however, they are best avoided completely. Butter, being almost completely fat, contains virtually no milk proteins, which is what most people react to. If you do not have a pronounced allergy to dairy products you may find that butter doesn't cause you a problem.

Yeast, another common allergen, is present in many processed foods, either as bakers' yeast, used in breads and pastries, or in drinks as brewers' yeast. About one in five people produce antibodies against it. Yeast is not completely avoidable, because natural yeasts are present in many foods, such as fruits, and also in wine; however, it is best to minimise the amount you consume.

You can find out if you are intolerant to a food by taking a pinprick blood test using a home test kit (see Resources). This identifies exactly which foods your immune system attacks. Your system does this by producing antibodies to the perceived threat, which are then detectable in the blood. In any case, our recipes minimise the use of wheat, milk and yeast, giving alternatives for those who are intolerant to these foods.

Good foods that can be hard to digest

Some foods, although inherently good for you, are hard for some people to digest. These include beans, lentils and chickpeas, as well as the cruciferous vegetables, cabbage, cauliflower, broccoli, Brussels sprouts and kale. If these foods make you bloat or give you

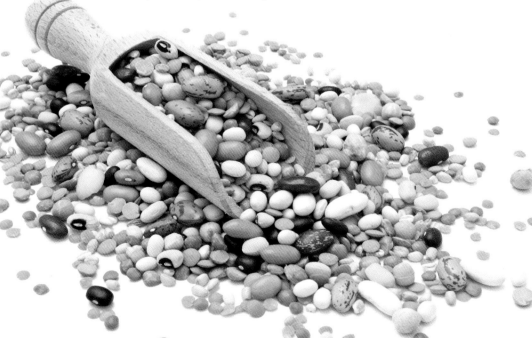

flatulence, you may be lacking an enzyme that helps you digest them and may need a little extra assistance. This is not an allergy but an enzyme deficiency. For beans you need an enzyme called alpha-galactosidase, while for greens you need an enzyme called amyloglucosidase. By taking a digestive enzyme supplement that contains these you may experience less bloating or flatulence when you eat these otherwise healthy foods.

Seeds and beans often have a coating that is indigestible, so that they can germinate after they have been digested by animals or birds. By cooking beans and lentils in the correct way, and rinsing them once or twice during the cooking process, you will help to break down these digestion inhibitors. The Chinese learned to ferment soya beans to achieve the same effect.

Even something as simple as grinding seeds will make them more digestible. All these foods are highly nutritious, because any seed food has to contain all the nutrients necessary for it to grow. Also, wholefoods naturally contain the nutrients that help your body to not only digest food, but also to use the key nutrients in food for energy or cell regeneration.

Tips for digestion-friendly habits and foods

- Don't eat when you are stressed – stress inhibits digestion.
- Chew your food well. This makes a big difference, because the enzymes in saliva help to break carbohydrates down. So ensure you chew your food until the particles are broken down.
- Eat foods raw or as lightly cooked as possible.
- Eat whole foods that naturally contain the nutrients needed for their digestion.
- Eat soft fruits (such as melons, peaches and berries), which break down easily, as snacks, not as desserts after a protein-rich meal. Protein takes longer to digest and soft fruits can ferment in the digestive tract.
- Either avoid or reduce wheat, milk or yeast (found in beer but not spirits, bread but not pasta) or, ideally, test what you're allergic to (see Resources). (The menus allow for a maximum of one serving of wheat or milk or a food containing yeast, with plenty of options that are completely free from these foods.)

2: Eat a low-GL diet, lose weight and gain energy

To be 100 per cent healthy you need to become a master of your blood sugar balance, because your body relies on a steady and even blood sugar level. As a consequence of mastering your blood sugar balance you will feel full of energy, you'll stop craving sugar and stimulants – and you'll lose weight and keep it off. In contrast, blood sugar that is out of kilter causes weight gain and ill health.

Glucose is the main energy-giving fuel for the body and brain, and keeping your blood glucose level as even as possible is not only the secret to having high mental and physical energy but it also protects you from the ever-increasing list of common health problems listed below.

Keeping your blood sugar level even can help prevent…

• Cancer
• Heart disease and strokes
• Diabetes and sugar cravings
• Weight gain, especially around the middle
• Polycystic ovaries and PMS
• Low mood, poor memory and, ultimately, Alzheimer's disease
• Liver damage, gout, psoriasis and many more common ailments

Achieving an even blood sugar level

The question is, how do you keep your blood sugar even? By definition a meal that achieves this vital goal is called 'low GL', with GL standing for glycemic load. The GL of a food is an accurate indicator of the impact of a particular food or meal on your blood sugar. The higher the GL the greater the impact. A meal with a low GL will be made up of a type of carbohydrate that contains slow-releasing sugars (called low GI, or glycemic index) and a larger portion of protein, because protein takes longer to digest and hence slows down the release of carbohydrates from the digestive tract into the blood. Eating such meals 'little and often' further helps to maintain an even blood sugar level.

How to keep your blood sugar even

Always eat breakfast, lunch and dinner – and introduce a snack mid morning and mid afternoon. This way you'll provide your body with a constant and even supply of fuel, which means you'll experience fewer food cravings. You also need to cut back on stimulants, particularly if you are in the habit of drinking coffee with a carbohydrate snack, such as a croissant. According to research at Canada's University of Guelph, this is a deadly duo as far as your blood sugar is concerned. Participants were given a carbohydrate snack, such as a croissant, muffin or toast, together with either a decaf or coffee. Those having the coffee–carb combo had triple the increase in blood sugar levels, while insulin sensitivity was almost halved. The odd coffee, on it's own, is not a major health problem as far as disease risk is concerned; however, in our survey, those who consumed no caffeinated drinks had almost twice the chance (11 per cent) of being in optimal health compared to those consuming one to two a day (6 per cent).

The reason why peaks and troughs in your blood sugar level are to be avoided at all costs is that the peaks lead to more insulin release, which effectively opens up the gates in the arteries to dump excess sugar into the liver, where it is promptly turned into fat, usually around your middle. The more often this happens, the more 'resistant' or insensitive you become to the hormone insulin, forcing the body to make even more. The resulting higher levels of blood glucose, and insulin, are what increase the risk of all those diseases listed earlier.

Also, peaks in blood sugar levels often lead to troughs, as too much insulin kicks in too late. This leads to a low blood sugar level, with corresponding energy dips, tiredness, grumpiness, sleepiness and poor concentration.

How many GLs should you aim for?

As I pointed out earlier, the glycemic load (GL) of a food tells you the effect that food will have on your blood sugar, and because fluctuations in blood sugar levels point to increases in weight, it's the best way of telling you which foods to avoid or to eat less of if you want to lose weight or to maintain a healthy weight. Foods and their quantities are given a GL value. To maintain your weight, most people need to eat 60GLs a day, and to lose weight they need to eat no more than 40GLs a day. There's a further 5GLs a day for drinks or snacks, bringing the total to 45 (or 65GLs a day for maintenance). (This is explained in detail in my *Low-GL Diet Bible*, which provides day-to-day guidelines to help you lose the maximum amount of weight without going hungry.)

To lose weight, this means 10GLs for breakfast, lunch and dinner, and two 5GL snacks. For maintenance, this means 15GLs per main meal and 7.5GLs per snack.

The main meals in this book are all devised to average out at around 10GLs, which is perfect if you want to lose weight. If you simply want to maintain your weight, you can just slightly increase the portion size of any carbohydrate accompaniment like pasta, potatoes or rice. We have given you portion sizes for carbohydrates on page 81. The total GL of a meal on a maintenance diet should be around 15.

For those without significant weight issues, almost any combination of these recipes is going to be broadly consistent with a low-GL diet, although we give you daily menus that achieve that perfect balance throughout the day. For those wanting to maximise weight loss you can choose the lower GL recipes, and appropriate variations in serving sizes, to equate to the total of 45GLs a day.

The rules of GL balance

There are four golden rules for keeping your blood sugar level even:

Rule 1 Eat 40 GL s a day to lose weight, 60 to maintain it.

Rule 2 Eat carbohydrate with protein.

Rule 3 Graze, don't gorge, eating little and often.

Rule 4 Cut back on stimulants.

The best low-GL foods

The main criteria that make a food low GL is (a) how much carbohydrate it contains; (b) what specific kind of carbohydrate or sugar it is made out of, including indigestible fibre – especially soluble fibres such as in oats, which help to slow down the release of the sugars in a food; and (c) how much protein is in the food. Beans and lentils, for example, contain slow-releasing carbohydrates, fibres and protein, and hence are very low GL. In this context, beans instead of potatoes with a main meal would have a big effect in lowering the GL of the meal.

Berries, cherries and plums contain a type of sugar, called xylose, which is very slow releasing, whereas bananas, dates and raisins provide fast-releasing glucose. Apples and pears, containing fructose, are somewhere in the middle. Each of these foods, in their natural state, contain fibre, further lowering their GL, but juices have the fibre removed and are therefore higher GL.

Grains, being predominantly carbohydrate, are higher GL, but oats, which contain more protein and soluble fibre, are much lower GL than wheat. The more refined the food the higher the GL, so white rice is higher than brown rice. (Brown rice tastes better and has a slightly nutty flavour, but it takes longer to cook than white rice.) Brown rice also expands more because it contains more water-absorbing fibres. This means that brown rice and other low-GL cereals make you feel fuller for longer.

You can a find list of the GL values of foods in my books *The Low-GL Diet Bible* and *The 10 Secrets of 100% Healthy People* or in the pocket guide book *The Low-GL Diet Counter* – or look at the online version on www.holforddiet.com. But you don't need to have them to use this cookbook. For these recipes we have selected low-GL ingredients so that you don't have to concern yourself with looking up lists, but if you want to 'do it yourself' and concoct your own low-GL recipes the lists will give you the knowledge to branch out.

Eat protein with carbohydrate

The other principle we apply in the recipes and menus is to always combine protein with carbohydrate; for example, beans or fish and rice, such as the Lentil Dahl with rice on page 153, or meat with a root vegetable mash, like Shepherd's Pie with Sweet Potato Topping on page 127, or the Porridge with Almonds and Goji Berries on page 89. This simple rule is easy to develop into a habit. Any 'seed' food, such as beans, lentils, chickpeas, nuts or seeds, is essential protein that is as rich as animal produce, except for milk.

Since protein takes much longer to digest than carbohydrate – because it slows down the action of emptying of the stomach contents into the intestines – eating more protein and less carbohydrate immediately lowers the GL of a meal. This effect happens because protein is more acidic than carbohydrate, so until the stomach acid has worked on the protein, the carbohydrates, which require a more alkaline intestinal environment, cannot be digested. Other ways of increasing the acidity of the stomach include squeezing lemon or lime juice over a meal, or vinegar, perhaps in a salad dressing.

We have applied these principles in the daily menus, and most of the individual recipes, to give you a low-GL meal that effortlessly makes you feel fuller and more satisfied for longer.

Tips for a low-GL diet

- Don't eat more than 60GLs per day in total, aiming for main meals of 10–15GLs and a snacks or light meals of up to 7.5GLs. Each recipe has a GL score.
- Make low-GL foods, such as oats and pulses (beans, lentils, chickpeas), berries, cherries and plums, staple foods in your diet.
- Eat fruit – don't drink it.
- Eat three main meals and two snacks a day.
- Always combine protein and carbohydrate foods in a meal.
- Add lemon or lime juice and vinegar to your meals.

3: Improve your mood and memory with B vitamins

Have you ever wondered how your brain and body's chemistry manages to stay in balance? How does it make insulin when your blood sugar is high, or adrenalin when you're stressed – to name just two of thousands of vital 'communication' chemicals? And how does it break them down when balance is restored? Behind the scenes, every second of every day, there's a process called methylation that keeps just about everything in check. It's the key to feeling connected – happy, alert and motivated. It even helps you to eliminate fat, and it cuts your risk of just about every disease, as well as keeping your bones strong and stopping you from losing your memory.

How good you are at methylation is indicated by the level of a simple substance in your blood called homocysteine (see page 18), which is easily measured either by your GP or you can do it yourself using a home test kit (see Resources). Although 'homocysteine' doesn't exactly roll off the tongue, you need to commit it to memory, because your homocysteine, or H, score is your single most important health statistic. Keeping your homocysteine low, indicating that you are good at methylation and able to rapidly adapt and respond to life's stresses, is a secret of 100% Health. As the list below illustrates, this process is crucial.

Methylation, and hence your homocysteine, is vital for…

• Building bones – a high H score predicts osteoporosis.
• Copying DNA – a high H score predicts a higher risk of pregnancy problems.
• Repairing DNA – a high H score is associated with increased cancer risk.
• Preventing arterial damage – a high H score predicts an increased risk of heart attacks and strokes.
• Preventing brain damage – a high H score predicts a risk of depression, memory loss and Alzheimer's disease.
• Making neurotransmitters and cellular energy – neurotransmitters are linked to your energy level and your stress tolerance. A high H score suggests that your energy levels and stress tolerance level are low.

If you want to be 100 per cent healthy, and happy, you need to have a low homocysteine level, which means that you are good at methylation. But how do you achieve this? The 'cogs' of the methylation process are enzymes and these are dependent on a range of B vitamins and other nutrients, specifically:

B$_6$ Found in lentils, beans, nuts, seeds, meat, fish, greens and some fruits
Folic acid Found in lentils, beans, nuts, seeds, green vegetables and some fruits
B$_{12}$ Found in meat, fish, eggs, milk, nuts and seeds
Zinc Found in meat, fish, eggs, milk, nuts and seeds
TMG (tri-methyl-glycine) Found in eggs and root vegetables

Our recipes are designed and rated for their content of these methylation nutrients.

Improving your H score

Exactly how much of these key methylation nutrients you need depends on many factors, including your genes, your lifestyle, your age and your current state of health. Some people inherit an inability to build highly efficient methylation enzymes and therefore need more B vitamins as a result.

The older you are the less well you absorb vitamin B$_{12}$ but some people are born poor B$_{12}$ absorbers. That's why I always say that the best starting point is to measure your homocysteine level and, if it is above 7mmol/l, then you need to supplement these nutrients as well as eating a good diet. Exactly how much you need, depending on your homocysteine level, is explained in detail in *The 10 Secrets of 100% Healthy People*, which also gives you are in-depth understanding of the methylation process.

If you want to reverse one of the homocysteine-related disease processes, you will probably need to supplement much higher levels of these nutrients than you could possibly achieve with diet alone; as was found during research involving people who had age-related cognitive decline, and a corresponding homocysteine level of above 9. Supplements of 800mcg folic acid, 500mcg vitamin B$_{12}$ and 20mg of vitamin B$_6$ not only stopped memory decline and, for some, improved it, but it also arrested accelerated brain shrinkage, the hallmark of Alzheimer's disease. Although you could probably eat 400mcg of folic acid (found in leafy greens and pulses), you would be hard pushed to eat more than 5mcg of

B_{12}, which although found in animal produce is only one hundredth of the level shown to prevent your brain shrinking. The recommended daily allowance (RDA) given for vitamin B_{12}, which is the amount contained in most high-street vitamin supplements, is a mere 1mcg, but that is not nearly enough for people aged over 60.

The homocysteine-lowering diet

The best place to start is always with diet, which is why our recipes and menus include foods high in these nutrients. Although vitamin B_{12} is not so easy to increase in your diet (unless you eat tons of meat, which is not good for your health), you can increase folic acid by making good food choices. Folic acid, as its name suggests, is high in 'foliage' – as in green leafy vegetables, but you may be surprised to see that lentils, beans, nuts and seeds are just as good, if not better, as shown below.

The best foods for folate

Food	Amount per 100g (3½ oz) serving
Wheatgerm	325mcg
Lentils, cooked	179mcg
Millet flakes	170mcg
Sunflower seeds	164mcg
Endive	142mcg
Chickpeas, dried, cooked	141mcg
Spinach	140mcg
Romaine lettuce	135mcg
Broccoli	130mcg
Kidney beans, dried, cooked	115mcg
Peanuts	110mcg
Brussels sprouts	110mcg
Orange juice, fresh or frozen	109mcg
Asparagus	98mccg
Hazelnuts	72mcg
Avocado	66mcg

Many of these foods are also good sources of vitamin B_6 and, in the case of beans, lentils, nuts and seeds, zinc as well. These foods need to become a regular part of your diet.

Does your diet contain enough nutrients?

The big myth that even the most reasonably health-conscious people believe is that their diet alone can, and does, provide enough of the nutrients I have been discussing above. Have a look at the food combinations below. You would need to eat the equivalent of any one of these a day to have achieved an optimal intake of folic acid (called folate in food). Our menus aim to achieve this much using nutrient-rich foods that support optimal methylation.

Examples of what to eat to achieve 400mcg of folate

• A salad with Romaine lettuce, endive, half an avocado and a handful of sunflower seeds, accompanied by a glass of orange juice.

• A dish made with a serving of lentils or millet, with a serving each of spinach, broccoli and parsnips.

• A fruit salad with papaya, kiwi fruit, orange and cantaloupe melon in orange juice, plus a handful of unsalted peanuts.

• An orange, a large serving of broccoli, spinach, Brussels sprouts and a bowl of miso soup.

The symbol for B vitamins

Folic acid is just one of the important methylation B vitamins. To make sure you get a good amount of B vitamins to aid methylation, we have rated the recipes on a scale of one to three, using the symbol $\boxed{\text{B}}$. One $\boxed{\text{B}}$ is scored if a dish contains vegetables, nuts or seeds, which are good sources of vitamins, including B_6. Similarly one $\boxed{\text{B}}$ is scored if a dish contains fish, meat, eggs or milk, which all provide vitamin B_{12}. Two $\boxed{\text{B}}$s are scored if a dish contains beans and pulses, which are particularly rich in folate. If a dish contains two types of vegetable and eggs, for example, then it scores three B̄s. You want to achieve three B̄s every day. So, if you have one recipe with 'B̄' and another with 'B̄ B̄' you've done it. If you want to achieve this easily at home, eat seven servings of fruit and vegetables a day, with plenty of methylation-boosting green vegetables and citrus fruit, have a small handful of raw nuts or seeds per day, and a portion of beans or lentils most days. Our daily menus achieve this.

Eating greens, and especially broccoli and other cruciferous vegetables, is especially important, because they are also rich sources of potent anti-cancer and detoxifying nutrients. (Cruciferous vegetables – whose leaves grow in a cross – include cabbage, cauliflower, kale and Brussels sprouts.) Broccoli is especially rich in I3C (Indole3carbonol), which mops up excess oestrogen, thereby reducing the risk of breast and prostate cancer.

In our 100% Health Survey those who ate five or more servings of vegetables daily were 40 per cent more likely to have an optimum health rating than those who did not eat vegetables. Also, those who ate nuts and seeds three or more times a day were 60 per cent more likely to have optimum health compared to those who didn't eat nuts and seeds. Although we didn't specifically look at bean and lentil intake, it is probable that intake of these foods will also be a good predictor of optimal health.

Tips to improve your mood and memory with B vitamins

- Aim for seven servings of fruit and vegetables a day; for example, fruit with breakfast and two fruit snacks, plus two servings of vegetables with each main meal.
- Eat plenty of green vegetables.
- Have a serving of beans or lentils most days.
- Have a small handful of raw nuts or seeds, perhaps ground on your breakfast cereal, or added to soups or as a snack with some fruit.

4: Increase the anti-ageing antioxidants

The process of ageing is largely determined by oxidation; that is, the gradual damage produced by the 'exhaust fumes' of burning the fuel in food – glucose – with oxygen. Oxygen is our most vital nutrient – without it we would die in minutes. Every cell depends on a steady supply of it, yet as we use it to extract the energy from food, we make oxidants, which damage not only our skin, which becomes less soft and flexible as a result, but also the membranes of all our cells, making them gradually less functional. The antidote to this process of ageing is to optimise your intake of nature's age defenders: antioxidants. These protect us from the DNA-damaging effects of oxidants.

Measuring food's antioxidant power

Foods high in antioxidants are naturally colourful – from yellow turmeric, to blueberries, orange carrots, red tomatoes and dark green vegetables such as broccoli – as in the colours of the rainbow. The different colours denote slightly different kinds of antioxidants, which in combination provide the most protection. Although colour is a good indication of the antioxidant power of a food, there is a more precise way to measure it using a food's ORAC (oxygen radical absorbency capacity) potential. This is an objective measure of how good a food is at dealing with the oxidant 'exhaust fumes' of life.

The oldest living communities consume at least 6,000 ORACs a day. Okinawa, an island off mainland Japan, for example, is home to one of the longest-living communities in the world. In a population of 1 million, there are 900 centenarians – four times more

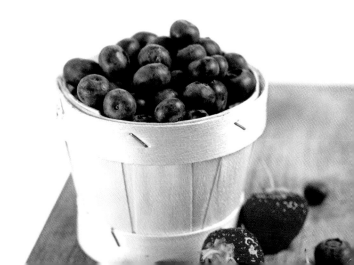

than in Britain and America. The Okinawans, in common with other peoples who enjoy a long life expectancy, include large amounts of antioxidant-rich fresh fruits and vegetables in their diets, and these prevent cell damage in the body. According to Dr Richard Cutler, former director of the US Government Anti-aging Research Department, 'the amount of antioxidants that you maintain in your body is directly proportional to how long you will live'.

6,000 ORACs a day keeps ageing at bay

The chart below shows the ORACs of 20 different foods that you can incorporate easily into your daily diet. Each serving contains approximately 2,000 units, so by choosing at least three of these daily you'll hit your anti-ageing score of 6,000:

1	⅓ tsp ground cinnamon	11	7 walnut halves
2	½ tsp dried oregano	12	8 pecan halves
3	½ tsp ground turmeric	13	¼ cup pistachio nuts
4	1 heaped tsp mustard	14	½ cup cooked lentils
5	⅕ cup blueberries	15	1 cup cooked kidney beans
6	½ pear, grapefruit or plum	16	⅓ medium avocado
7	½ cup blackcurrants, berries, raspberries or strawberries	17	½ cup red cabbage
8	½ cup cherries or a shot of Cherry Active concentrate	18	2 cups broccoli
9	1 orange or apple	19	1 medium artichoke or 8 asparagus spears
10	4 pieces of dark chocolate (70 per cent cocoa solids)	20	⅓ medium glass (150ml/5fl oz/ 1/4 pint) red wine

Source: Oxygen Radical Absorbance Capacity of Selected Foods – 2007, US Department of Agriculture

The symbols for ORAC content

Our daily menus aim to provide at least 6,000 ORACs a day. To make this simple for you we've assigned a symbol of a carrot to denote 1,000 ORACs. Whichever recipes you choose, make sure you get six 🥕 a day. Also, when you create your own menus, if you do choose multi-coloured ingredients, covering all the main colours in a day, the chances are you'll achieve the golden 6,000 ORACs (or 🥕🥕🥕🥕🥕🥕) guideline.

Berries, cherries and plums rule

Fruits that have the highest levels of ORACs are those with the deepest colour, such as blueberries, raspberries and strawberries. These are particularly rich in powerful antioxidants called anthocyanadins. One cup, 115g (4oz), of blueberries will provide 9,697 units. You would need to eat 11 bananas to get the same benefit as a cupful of blueberries! As you also saw earlier, berries are rich in xylose, which keeps your blood sugar level even, whereas bananas contain a lot of glucose and, unless you are exercising a lot, will promote abdominal weight gain.

One of the simplest and easiest ways to achieve a guaranteed 6,000 ORACs is to have a daily shot of a Montmorency cherry concentrate, called Cherry Active, diluted with water. This measures 8,260 on the ORAC scale, which is the equivalent of around 23 portions of regular fruit and vegetables! Other juices, such as acai and pomegranate, also claim high ORAC scores, but this tops the lot. You will see we have created some desserts that include a little Cherry Active or berries. We also use dark chocolate and cinnamon, both of which are exceptionally high in antioxidants.

Seven of the best

The amount of fruit and vegetables you need per day in order to meet your ORAC quota really does depend on which ones you choose, as you can see in the menus for two days below. Both days have five portions selected, but Day 2's selection is 8,000

Choose the 'best value' fruit and veg

DAY 1		DAY 2	
Fruit/vegetable portion	ORAC	Fruit/vegetable portion	ORAC
⅛ large cantaloupe melon	315	½ pear	2,617
Kiwi fruit	802	½ cup strawberries	2,683
1 medium carrot, raw	406	½ avocado	2,899
½ cup green peas, frozen	432	1 cup broccoli, raw	1,226
1 cup spinach, raw	455	4 asparagus spears, boiled	986
Total score	2,410	Total score	10,411

ORACs more than that for Day 1. However, if you aim for seven servings a day – that's three fruit servings and two vegetable servings with each main meal – you'll easily achieve 6,000 ORACs, or 🥕🥕🥕🥕🥕.

Reduce your oxidant exposure

The flip side of the antioxidant equation is to reduce your exposure to oxidants – that is 'burnt' oxygen. Smoking is an example, but so too is deep-frying or putting cheese on top of a dish and baking or grilling it to go crispy. Caramelising, which is burning sugar, is also bad news. Poaching, steam-frying and preparing dishes raw, only heating them to serve, are all ways of reducing oxidant exposure.

The kind of oil you cook with also makes a big difference. In the next section we'll discuss how to optimise your intake of essential fats, found principally in fish, nuts and seeds. Such essential fats are easily oxidised when heated, however, especially at high temperatures. So, when you sauté a food it is much better to use a source of fat or oil that is saturated, which means it would be solid, or almost solid, at room temperature. Butter, for example, or coconut butter are saturated fats. Olive oil, containing the mono-unsaturated fat called oleic acid, is close to saturated. Heating these oils creates much fewer oxidants. When a heated fat reaches its 'smoking point' then you are really generating a lot of oxidants.

Tips for increasing the anti-ageing antioxidants in your diet

- Eat multicoloured foods every day, aiming to eat foods from each of the different colour groups, from yellow and orange to red, green and purple.
- Have lots of herbs and spices.
- Aim for seven servings of fruit and vegetables per day.
- Choose daily menus that give you 🥕🥕🥕🥕🥕 per day.
- Keep frying to a minimum, choosing steam-frying, light stir-frying or poaching instead.
- Use butter, coconut butter, or olive oil or rapeseed oil for cooking.

5: Eat the essential fats

There are certain fats that your body needs in plenty and they are called 'essential fats', because they are necessary for the each cell to function properly. As you may know, your body is made largely of water. This is contained within cells that have a membrane made of essential fats. The membrane perceives changes in the environment outside the cell and then reacts accordingly. In this way, fats are part of how our cells 'perceive' and adapt. For many years, fat was believed to be something we must avoid eating for good health, but we now know that essential fats are vital for many processes in the body.

Essential fats are vital for…

• A good mood and motivation
• A sharp memory
• A strong immune system
• Hormonal balance
• Reducing the risk of heart disease, strokes, diabetes and cancer
• Keeping your skin velvety smooth and youthful
• Reducing pain and inflammation

Although larger supplemental amounts are needed to reverse disease processes – for example, if you have heart disease, arthritis or clinical depression – we all need a daily supply. As you can see in the diagram overleaf there are two main families of essential fats that we need: omega-6 and omega-3.

Omega-6 fats are made and stored in the seeds and nuts of hot-climate plants, such as sunflower and sesame.

Omega-3 fats are found in colder climate nut or seed oils, such as chia and flaxseeds, as well as walnuts. Pumpkin seeds contain a bit of both. Omega-3s are also richly present in cold-water plankton – the food of little fishes, and especially in oily fish.

The sources of omega-6 and -3 fats

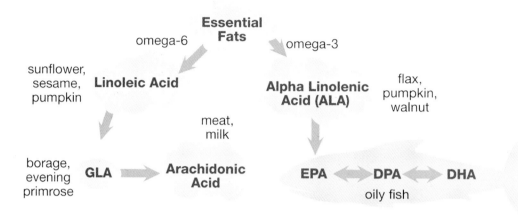

The most potent dietary source of omega-6 is called GLA, which is highly concentrated in evening primrose oil and borage oil. The most potent source of omega-3 is the trio of EPA, DPA and DHA, found only in significant quantities in oily or carnivorous fish (or in cod liver oil).

In effect, we are solar powered, relying on the plants we eat to store the sun's energy in carbohydrate, the body's primary fuel. Both vitamin D and essential fats are dependent on sunlight. Effectively, sunlight stored in plankton is passed up the food chain, through little fish into the carnivorous oily fish. In the case of seals, they eat the oily fish, and the oils are then stored in their fat and used as an energy source during the winter months – essential because they live in the darker regions of the world, which are devoid of sunlight for months on end. The Inuit survive, and stay healthy, in spite of their lack of sunlight, due to their high intake of nutrients in the seal meat they eat.

The decline in our oily fish consumption, largely because of a phobia of eating fat, has fuelled an epidemic in deficiencies of both omega-3 and vitamin D. This is doubly bad if you live far away from the equator – for example in the UK – with little strong sunlight and little desire to expose yourself to the sun's rays during the cold months of winter.

Getting the omega balance right

The further down the essential-fat chain you go, the more 'poly-unsaturated' the fat becomes, which makes it more biologically active, but also more prone to oxidative damage, which is what happens when an oil goes rancid. ALA, the vegetarian source of omega-3, is more prone to such damage than linoleic acid (omega-6). In the interests of making foods with a long shelf life, most processed foods have the omega-3 essential fats removed. As a consequence of this, plus with our fat phobia, we've ended up with a diet that is much more deficient in omega-3 than omega-6.

To be 100 per cent healthy you really want to focus on getting a source of omega-3 every day.

The best fish

Although it may not be environmentally correct, with declining levels of fish in the sea and an increasing population, the optimal intake of oily/carnivorous fish is three to five servings a week. The National Institute for Clinical Excellence (NICE) who advise NHS policy, recommend all heart-attack patients eat two to four portions of oily fish (herring, sardines, mackerel, salmon, tuna and trout) a week.

In our 100% Health Survey, we found that a person's chances of being in optimal health goes up by a third for those consuming three or more servings of oily fish a week, compared to two a week. A portion is defined as 140g (5oz), which is a small can of fish or a small fillet of fresh fish, from which one should derive at least 7g (⅛oz) of omega-3 essential fats over a week.

It is important to note, however, the level of omega-3s in canned tuna are a fraction of those in fresh. This is probably because the oil is often squeezed out, and may be sold to the supplement industry, leaving a drier meat disguised as such by then canning it in an inferior oil. In the US you can buy tuna in its own oil. It tastes completely different and much better. So, don't rely on canned tuna to provide your omega-3 quota, always try to use fresh fish. Another problem with oily fish is the potential for mercury contamination, particularly in very large fish such as tuna. This is particularly relevant for pregnant women, because mercury is a neurotoxin and can induce birth defects. I would recommend tuna once a fortnight during pregnancy and once a week or fortnight otherwise. The same advice applies to marlin or swordfish. The best all-rounders are probably wild salmon, mackerel and sardines. The level of omega-3s in farmed salmon depends on what they are fed.

Supplements and vegetarian sources of omega-3

Oily fish has health benefits unrelated to its omega-3 levels, being very high in protein, vitamin E, selenium and choline, from which we make tri-methyl glycine (TMG), a vital homocysteine-lowering nutrient. So I always advise eating three portions a week (but just don't count canned tuna!), but I also suggest supplementing as well, especially on those days that you don't eat fish.

The best vegetarian sources of omega-3 are chia seeds and flax seeds, followed by hemp seeds, pumpkin seeds and walnuts. Regarding pumpkin seeds, the colder the climate they grow in the more omega-3s they will contain. You also get some omega-3s in meat, dairy products, eggs from chickens fed on flax seeds, and cold-climate vegetables, such as kale, cabbage, broccoli, cauliflower and Brussels sprouts. Although this kind of omega-3 (ALA) is not as potent as the kind found in oily fish (EPA, DPA and DHA) some of it will be converted into these most potent forms.

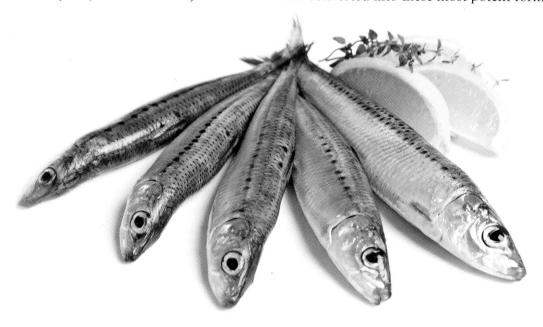

I like to eat a vegetarian source of omega-3s most days, my favourite being chia seeds. These taste delicious and are high in protein, essential fats and antioxidants, and are also a rich source of soluble fibres. Chia seeds were once a staple food in Central America, but the invading Spanish conquistadores, over 500 years ago, disliked the locals worshipping the seeds and so banned their cultivation. Only now are they making a comeback. Chia seeds are available in health-food stores and online (see Resources) and look like dark sesame seeds. Due to their size, they are best ground or soaked to maximise their absorption of nutrients. Next best are flax seeds.

The symbol for essential omegas

Our recipes are created with these essential omegas in mind. Any recipe that contains omega-3s is denoted with a Ω symbol. Your goal, for optimal health, is to achieve three Ω a day. One serving of oily fish gives you $\Omega\,\Omega\,\Omega$, whereas a serving of white fish gives you $\Omega\,\Omega$, and a tablespoon of chia or flax seeds, or a small handful of walnuts, gives you Ω. Our menus are designed to give you $\Omega\,\Omega\,\Omega$ a day.

Protect your omegas

As I explained in the last section, any cooking process using high heat will oxidise and destroy the value of these essential fats, so you want to eat your nuts and seeds raw and ideally poach, bake, lightly grill, steam-fry (described on page 71) or stir-fry oily fish. You don't want to eat burnt flesh as such. Smoked fish, such as salmon, is actually a slow-cook method and the fish itself is closer to raw fish and hence remains a good source of omega-3s.

Vital vitamin D

The other essential fat many of us are deficient in, especially during the winter, is vitamin D. Although you may know that it is essential for keeping your bones strong, this fat-based hormone does so much more. It may prove to be one of the most important cancer preventers, as well as being vital for a healthy nervous system – and hence brain function

– and as a good all-round immune-booster. Low levels of vitamin D in the winter months may be one of the reasons why we become more susceptible to colds.

The importance of vitamin D, beyond its role in bone health, was noticed when researchers investigated possible reasons why the prevalence of a number of diseases, including many forms of cancer, MS and schizophrenia, increased in relation to the distance people live from the equator.

The minimum level we need for optimal health is around 30mcg a day, although some experts say this is too low. If you expose yourself to moderate sunlight for 30 minutes a day and eat eggs and oily fish such as mackerel, you might achieve 15mcg. From November to February, however, it is unlikely you'll get enough high-intensity sun exposure to make even this if you live in more northerly areas. Hence, it is wise to supplement 15mcg, especially if you live in the UK or another country the equivalent distance from the equator or further away. You'll find this quantity in a good, high-strength multivitamin.

The best dietary source by a long way is oily fish, followed by eggs. I make a point of eating at least three servings of oily fish a week, plus at least six eggs which, by the way, won't increase your risk of heart disease or raise your blood cholesterol levels.

Tips for eating the essential fats

- Aim to have at least three servings of unfried oily fish (salmon, mackerel, herring, kipper, fresh tuna) a week, and four or more servings of fish a week.
- Eat some omega-3-rich raw seeds or nuts every day – a tablespoon of chia or flax seeds, or a small handful of walnuts or pumpkin seeds. If you are a strict vegetarian or vegan you'll need double this amount.
- Have at least six free-range or organic eggs a week, preferably from chickens fed with omega-3s (such as flax seeds).
- Expose yourself to at least 30 minutes of sunlight every day, when possible.

6: Drink enough water to keep yourself hydrated

It is an amazing fact that two-thirds of your body is water. Your brain is actually 85 per cent water. Yet, we take water, as a nutrient, for granted. If you become thirsty you drink – end of story, but most of us don't drink enough and don't eat sufficient fresh foods with a high water content. Two common consequences are constipation and fatigue.

How much do you really need?

The average man needs between 1.2 litres (2 pints) and 3 litres (5¼ pints) per day, whereas a woman needs between 1.2 litres (2 pints) and 2.2 litres (3¾ pints) – that averages out at about eight glasses or more of water-based liquid a day. We get about 19 per cent of our requirement from the food we eat, with fresh fruit and vegetables containing the most. So, the more fruit and veg you eat the more water you take in. Conversely, concentrated foods with a high sugar or protein content increase your need for water to dilute the excess sugars or break down the products of amino acids in the bloodstream.

Dehydration is defined as a 1 per cent or greater loss of body weight as a result of fluid loss; however, we feel thirsty when dehydration reaches 0.8–2 per cent. In other words, you can be dehydrated (you have lost over 1 per cent of your body weight) but not yet feel thirsty.

Drinking affects how much we eat

Because it's easy to think we are hungry when in fact we are thirsty, many of us eat instead of drinking to satisfy the sense of lack. However, there is some evidence that either drinking water with a meal or eating water-rich foods, such as fruit and veg, makes you likely to eat less. Water may also increase your metabolism in such a way that could encourage weight loss.

Your body retains much more if you drink little and often, rather than having it all in one go. Also, if water is drunk with sugar, which is so often the case in sugary drinks, the water is less well retained by the body. This will also be the case if drunk in tea or coffee.

There is nothing better than water. It satisfies your thirst and has no calories. So, if you are thirsty, the best thing is to drink a glass of water – and you can actually make the water you drink help you lose weight and stabilise your blood sugar by combining it with food.

'Eating' water

One of the triggers for controlling appetite is stomach extension. If your meal contains plenty of fibre-rich foods and is prepared in such a way that the fibre absorbs water and is bulkier, this makes the stomach more extended. If two people eat exactly the same food, one with a glass of water and the other with the glass of water added to their food – for example, by turning the meal into soup – the latter feels more full, because the stomach expands more. So, puréed soups are good news for appetite control. The water of the water-drinker quickly passes through the stomach. This also means that soaking your oats, or having porridge is likely to make you feel fuller than simply pouring milk on cereal. We use these principles in our recipes to maximise your water intake.

Whatever you do, make sure that you are drinking the equivalent of eight glasses of water a day, which includes herb teas and the water you add to your food. Often thirst is confused with hunger so, before you eat, have a glass of water, and, while you eat, continue to sip a glass of water.

Tips for drinking enough water to keep yourself hydrated

- Drink, or add to the food you eat, the equivalent of eight glasses of water. This includes hot drinks.
- Drink little and often, throughout the day.
- Have plenty of fresh fruit and vegetables, which are naturally high in water.
- Have plenty of soups, broths and other high-water foods. These are included in our recipes and daily menus.

7: Let food keep you fit

In our 100% Health Survey, 92 per cent of the top health scorers considered themselves to be moderately fit. There are two parts to keeping physically fit. The first is doing the correct kind and amount of exercise, and the second is eating the right foods. Protein is an essential food, because the amino acids contained therein are needed for boosting your mood and motivation, and for maintaining muscle mass. The older you become the more your muscle mass tends to decrease unless you consciously exercise and increase your protein intake. (For advice on the best kind of exercise to do, see *The 10 Secrets of 100% Healthy People.*)

Are you eating enough protein?

The amount of protein you need depends on how much exercise you are taking. Resistance exercise builds muscle; this is any exercise that stresses muscles to the point of some strain. Holding a yoga pose, practising Pilates or lifting a weight, are classic examples. Short-term stresses on muscles stimulate their growth and repair, which demands protein.

Any seed food that would grow into a plant contains protein. So, nuts, seeds, beans, lentils and chickpeas are all protein, as is quinoa. So too are eggs (the 'seed' of the chicken), poultry, meat and fish.

Grains contain their seed or germ, as in wheatgerm, surrounded by carbohydrate. The highest protein grain is oats. It is good to have some protein with every meal. So, for example, if you eat porridge oats and then add some chia or pumpkin seeds, and pour over soya milk, each of these provide good-quality protein.

One of the golden rules for low-GL eating, discussed earlier, is to combine protein with carbohydrate at each meal. Coupled with some resistance exercise, this is a great way to increase your muscle mass. Resistance exercise stimulates the natural release of growth hormone which helps increase lean muscle mass and this, in turn, burns fat.

How big is a protein serving?

Food	Weight	Which is approximately…
Tofu and tempeh	160g (5¾oz)	¾ packet
Soya mince	100g (3½oz)	3 tbsp
Chicken (no skin)	50g (1¾oz)	1 very small breast
Turkey (no skin)	50g (1¾oz)	½ small breast
Quorn	120g (4¼oz)	⅓ pack
Salmon and trout	55g (2oz)	1 very small fillet
Tuna (canned in brine)	50g (1¾oz)	¼ can
Sardines (canned in brine)	75g (2¾oz)	⅔ can
Cod	65g (2¼oz)	1 very small fillet
Clams	60g (2⅛ oz)	¼ can
Prawns	85g (3oz)	6 large prawns
Mackerel	85g (3oz)	1 medium fillet
Oysters	–	15
Yogurt (natural, low fat)	285g (10oz)	½ large tub
Cottage cheese	120g (4¼oz)	½ medium tub
Hummus	200g (7oz)	1 small tub
Skimmed milk	440ml	about 15fl oz/¾ pint
Soya milk	415ml	about 15fl oz/¾ pint
Eggs (boiled)	–	2
Quinoa	125g (4½oz)	large serving bowl
Baked beans	310g (11oz)	¾ can
Kidney beans	175g (6oz)	⅓ can
Black-eye beans	175g (6oz)	⅓ can
Lentils	165g (5¾oz)	⅓ can
Pumpkin seeds	52g (1¾oz)	heaped tbsp
Chia seeds	55g (2oz)	heaped tbsp
Almonds	82g (3oz)	¾ cup
Peanuts	67g (2¼oz)	½ cup

You need about 60g (2oz) of protein a day if you are exercising on a regular basis, including resistance training. You'll get some protein in your snacks, and also in the vegetable and carbohydrate portion of a meal – for example, oats and broccoli provide a reasonable amount of protein, so if you aim for a 15g (½oz) serving of a protein-rich food in a meal you'll be on the right track. Note, that's the weight of protein not the weight of the food. For a top quality vegetarian food, such as quinoa or beans, you'll need four times this quantity since around a quarter will be protein. For an animal or fish protein, you'll need twice as much since most fish and meat is half to two-thirds protein. The table opposite shows what you need to eat to achieve the target. It doesn't matter if you have a little more. By skewing your diet towards fish and vegetable protein you'll naturally be eating less saturated fats.

Our recipes and daily menus naturally give you a good supply of protein throughout the day so you do not need to calculate or monitor your protein quantities if you follow the menus and guidelines.

Aerobic exercise increases your nutrient needs

The other side of the exercise equation is to keep aerobically fit with some kind of endurance exercise that gets you puffing. This could be a good walk, especially if it involves walking uphill some of the time, a jog, a swim, a cycle or an aerobics-style class. The more aerobic-type exercise you do the more antioxidants you will need for dealing with the 'exhaust' fumes created by exercise. Muscles also use B vitamins (see page 30) to generate energy and the correct balance of calcium and magnesium is needed for muscles to contract and relax. Magnesium is commonly deficient in the modern diet but the recipes you find here contain plenty of nuts, seeds, beans, lentils and greens – all of which are great sources of magnesium.

Eat after exercise

From an evolutionary point of view, animals don't eat before exercise. They usually lie around until they are hungry, and then go hunting for food. Having successfully hunted they eat and then rest.

After exercise, the body's metabolism is hyped up and ready to eat. So, for example, if you exercise before breakfast, and then eat, you'll stay lean and healthy. The only time when this pattern becomes a problem is if you've already developed blood sugar problems, diabetes being the extreme, in which case you'll wake up with your blood sugar level too low and will crave something sweet or a stimulant drink. Under these circumstances, I recommend a small amount of fruit. This is also not a bad idea if you are going for a long walk or jog as it will keep your energy level up.

Gentle exercise helps your digestion, and taking some exercise also helps with appetite control. People who do no exercise tend to eat more than those with moderate exercise levels. Going for a stroll around the park after your Sunday lunch, then coming back and eating dessert is a good example of putting these principles into action.

Tips for keeping fit with food

- Eat protein with each meal, aiming for a 15g (½oz) protein food serving (that's the weight of protein, not the weight of the food).
- Combine protein with carbohydrate.
- Increase your intake of nutrient-rich foods, and take daily supplements providing B vitamins, antioxidants and magnesium, if you are doing endurance or aerobic exercise.
- Generally, eat after exercise, not before.

8: Choose high-vitality foods

Food is literally our source of energy, but which foods give you the most vitality? Oriental medicine has a whole tradition of not only eating foods with high vitality but also eating 'yin' and 'yang' foods to balance one's energy. Yang foods, such as meat, give you more active, aggressive energy, whereas 'yin' foods, such as fruits and vegetables, are associated with a more passive, receptive energy.

This roughly parallels another concept of balancing acid-forming foods – which are those high in protein, itself made from amino acids – with alkaline-forming foods, which are those that are naturally high in the alkaline minerals potassium, calcium, magnesium and sodium. Broadly speaking, the alkaline foods are fruits and vegetables. Although it is true that the body's clever chemistry works hard to maintain the same pH balance in the blood, if you eat too many acid-forming foods the blood's pH does become a little higher.

These alkaline minerals are also vital for the nervous system and muscles, and not getting enough magnesium, which is commonly deficient in the Western diet, does lead to both more anxiety and more muscle cramps. A number of studies show that taking in extra magnesium helps sleep, helps relax muscles and also lowers blood pressure. So, the idea of eating more alkaline-forming foods, and fewer acid-forming foods is consistent with being healthier.

Many vegetarian sources of protein, such as nuts, seeds, beans and the 'superfoods', such as quinoa and chia seeds, are also rich sources of alkaline minerals, which balance their concentration of amino acids. Hence, the idea of eating more vegetarian sources of protein fits in as well.

Raw food energy

Almost any form of cooking is going to destroy the nutrients in foods. The higher the temperature and the longer the cooking, the more nutrients are destroyed. Boiling vegetables for too long, for example, causes greater losses of water-soluble B and C vitamins, whereas frying destroys fat-soluble vitamin E and essential fats. Cooking can also break down proteins and, since natural enzymes within certain foods are proteins, it may make some foods less digestible.

You will benefit from the most nutrients in food by eating as much of your food as raw as possible. Cooking methods such as steam-frying (see page 71) doesn't lead to much nutrient loss. The same is true for steaming or poaching food for a few minutes. At least, if you make something like a soup you are consuming the water, in which some of the nutrients will remain. You can also make soups cold, and heat to serve if necessary (for example the Raw Red Pepper and Tomato Soup on page 106). Many of our recipes are designed to minimise nutrient losses in this way.

Solar-powered first-class food

We literally derive our energy from the sun. Plants use the sun's energy to make carbohydrate, forming the body of the plant, derived from the basic elements of carbon, hydrogen and oxygen, which are captured from the earth and water, and from converting carbon dioxide in the air into oxygen. Plants, just like us, are made from the fundamental elements of earth, water, air and the fire of the sun.

It makes sense that eating raw plants would be more energising than eating processed food. If a plant grows, and is cooked, and the scraps are fed to an animal, perhaps a pig, which is then killed, and its meat cooked, the end result is four times removed from the original plant. If a food is extensively cooked and processed, refined and artificially flavoured, then that would be even more denatured.

So, the golden rule is to only buy, or eat, foods that could be pulled out of the ground or out of a tree and, in relation to animal produce, to only eat animals that are fed pure, and not processed food; for example, a fish caught in unpolluted water, eaten fresh and raw (such as sushi), would be closest to natural food.

Of course, there are benefits in cooking some foods; for example, cooking meat reduces the risk of infection from bacteria in the meat. Many fish, especially the less healthy ones,

Vitality in foods

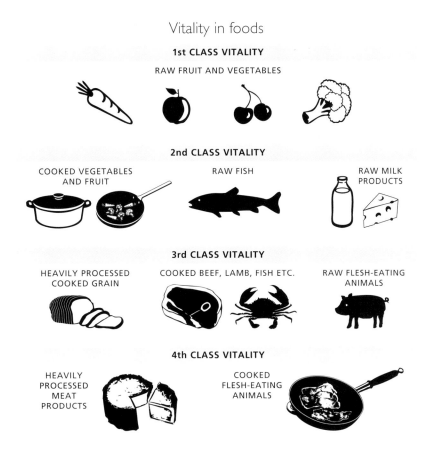

1st CLASS VITALITY

RAW FRUIT AND VEGETABLES

2nd CLASS VITALITY

COOKED VEGETABLES AND FRUIT   RAW FISH   RAW MILK PRODUCTS

3rd CLASS VITALITY

HEAVILY PROCESSED COOKED GRAIN   COOKED BEEF, LAMB, FISH ETC.   RAW FLESH-EATING ANIMALS

4th CLASS VITALITY

HEAVILY PROCESSED MEAT PRODUCTS   COOKED FLESH-EATING ANIMALS

contain parasites and there's a valid concern about the dangers of infection from eating too much raw fish. In days of old, when organic food wasn't so readily available (and in countries such as India where amoebic dysentery is a real concern), cooking methods such as deep-frying and extensive boiling developed to destroy the dangerous amoebas, but they also destroyed as many nutrients. This is not so necessary these days, if you have access to organic food or, better still, if you are able to grow your own vegetables.

Keep it natural, organic and whole

We have certainly moved a long way away from traditional, and healthier, farming practices during the last 50 years or so when all food was organic simply because pesticides and herbicides didn't exist. This is graphically illustrated in the film, *Food Inc*, which shows how far modern agriculture and food production has changed from the pre-war conception of 'farming'. Although worthwhile arguments are made for modern food-production methods being the only way we can feed our vastly expanding population, the fact is that modern man is getting sicker not healthier, and this really suggests that we are sacrificing quality for quantity, which is often really a synonym for profit.

It is ironic that you often have to pay more for foods that are unprocessed, such as brown rice. Organic foods often cost 25 per cent more, but they also contain more actual food, as well as nutrients, since most organic food contains less water than commercially grown food (a higher water content is an intentional by-product of fast-growing methods for producing higher yields). The important point to remember is that you are worth feeding well. Your body, and brain, are literally made from the food you eat, so don't skimp on the quality of the food you buy.

Tips for choosing high-vitality foods

- Aim to eat half your diet as raw food and at least two-thirds as raw or lightly cooked, steamed or stir-fried food.
- When you go shopping, the majority of what you buy should be fresh, whole food, not processed or pre-prepared food.
- Be mindful of any animal produce – fish, eggs, meat and milk – and make sure you only buy produce in which the animal has been fed the most natural food, organic if possible, and reared in a natural environment.
- Eat only whole grains, not white rice, pasta, bread and other denatured foods.
- Eat only raw nuts and seeds, not roasted and salted.
- Buy organic produce whenever you can, and grow your own herbs if possible.
- Stay away from processed foods, particularly foods with long lists of chemical additives and a seemingly indefinite shelf life.
- Have more alkaline-forming foods (fruit and vegetables) than acid-forming foods such as meat. Having more vegetable-based proteins, such as beans, lentils, chickpeas, quinoa, seeds and nuts, is a good way to angle your diet towards more alkaline foods.

9: Improve your relationship with food

One of the findings in our 100% Health Survey was the importance of good relationships for health. Among the healthiest people in our survey the vast majority had a positive attitude and 95 per cent considered relationships to be very important for overall health. This includes your relationship to food.

Food is much more than the means for physical nourishment. It can also be used almost as a drug, stimulating endorphins and dopamine – the very same pathways stimulated by heroin and cocaine, which literally make you feel high. In many Western cultures food has almost become the new sex, with endless new restaurants, cookbooks, TV programmes and other obsessions focused around culinary delights. And why not, provided the food is good and keeps you healthy?

In contrast, food, especially in excess, can be used to numb pain. Partly, this is learned behaviour that goes back to childhood. Perhaps, when you were a child and hurt yourself your mother consoled you with something sweet. Partly it is physiological; for example, eating something sweet does tend to improve your mood, because the mood-boosting neurotransmitter, serotonin, requires insulin to be transported into the brain. Both the psychological expectation of relief and the physiological effect flood the body with a cascade of 'reward' signals, making you feel good. In excess, however, both sugar and food in general start to create a numbing effect, a bit like being drunk. Then, you either don't have the energy or you can't quite think about what it was that was bothering you. This, plus a couple of glasses of wine, is our most popular way to forget about life's daily stresses.

The love–hate relationship with food

We can also have negative associations with food. For many people, food is a friend because it feels comforting to eat but an enemy as the pounds creep on, causing unattractive changes in body shape and with increasing health problems in close pursuit. As the weight piles on, those health problems can become life threatening, including diabetes, heart disease and even cancer. In fact, being obese accounts for increasing the risk of cancer in women by 20 per cent, whereas smoking increases the risk by 30 per cent. But while in the grip of this love–hate relationship with food, many people become food fanatics or are embroiled in food phobias or fads, strictly avoiding all fats, or all carbs, and frequently going from one diet extreme to another. What is more, certain foods, and especially sugar, milk and wheat, have an opioid-like effect; in the case of sugar you can literally become addicted to it. Then there are the stimulants, such as caffeine in caffeinated drinks, coffee and chocolate (which also contains the addictive compound theobromine). These feed an addictive relationship to those foods.

What is you relationship with food? Think carefully about the questions below and note down your answers. This can help you identify if you have any emotionally charged issues with food.

Questionnaire: what is your relationship with food?

1. Are there any foods you really dislike? What is your first memory of this food? Was it a bad one? Write down the food and your first negative memory of it.

2. Which foods do you think you shouldn't eat but you adore?

3. Which foods do you like eating but don't like the after effects?

4. What foods do you think you should eat, but don't really like that much?

5. Which foods or drinks would you find really hard to quit for a week? When did you last do it and for how long?

6. Are there any foods you have purposely avoided for a week or more? If so, write down those foods.

7. Do you find cooking:

   a) a chore?

   b) a pleasure?

   c) something in between?

8. Do you feel incompetent as a cook?

9. Do you enjoy making new dishes?

Once you have recognised which unhealthy foods you binge on or eat in excess, you can start to break those habits by not keeping those particular foods in the house. Reward yourself by eating healthy alternatives at appropriate times. Healthy snacking is good as long as you stick to the overall regime outlined in the recipe section, and you will also find some tempting snack ideas there. For healthy foods that you have an aversion, introduce small quantities into other foods and really taste the flavour, as a pure flavour rather than with a preconceived prejudice. You may find you start to like it. Babies need to taste a new food up to fifteen times before they like it. You may also find that once you widen your repertoire of foods you will get so much more enjoyment out of eating that you won't be drawn to the unhealthy foods in the same way.

Nurturing yourself through home-cooked food

Nowadays, we spend much less of our overall budget on our food shopping, and much more on eating out. Generally, there is less time and priority given to preparing meals, and many people have never learned the basic skills passed down from generation to generation. All of these factors, together with our accumulated emotional charge, can contribute to a worsening relationship with food. At it's extreme this can lead to eating disorders such as anorexia, bulimia and food addiction.

The purpose of this cookbook is to cut through some of this emotional clutter and give you relatively simple and delicious meals to prepare that tick the boxes for what your body really needs. The effect is that you will feel better relatively quickly and, over several weeks, you will generate a sense of well-being that acts as a reward to keep you going while, hopefully, hard-wiring some of these new eating habits. The recipes will introduce you to new foods, and new ways of preparing dishes with staple foods. It's good to experiment with new foods, expanding your repertoire, and you will have the pleasure of knowing that the simple meals you have prepared are really good for you.

Rome wasn't built in a day

My recommendation is that you follow the guidelines listed in this section for six days out of seven, giving yourself one day off, and also allow yourself two meal or snack deviations during the week on the condition that you record what prompted the deviation. Keep a diary or notebook with the following headings:

Date:
....

Food deviation   Feeling before   Feeling after   Consequences

This will help you identify any problem areas, such as a mid-afternoon slump or periods of stress. You can then take action to deal with them in another way that doesn't have negative consequences like weight gain, such as popping out for a break or ringing a friend.

Meals are important

How you eat, and who you eat with, are also important. Eating on the move, while working or watching TV has contributed to less fulfilling relationships, both with food and with family and friends. It is also better to eat when you are not stressed, because the net effect of the stress hormones, adrenalin and cortisol, is to shut down digestion. A simple act of preparing a meal, or meeting a friend for lunch, can give you a much-needed break in a stressful day.

There are lots of studies that show that families who eat together have more fulfilling relationships. The same is true with couples who make an effort to cook meals for each other, or together. How often do you do this?

Dealing with temptations and peer pressure

Although you may decide to eat in a certain way, perhaps avoiding a food such as milk, wheat or meat, or giving alcohol a break for a couple of weeks, this can sometimes become harder to do when you eat out or socialise with friends or work colleagues.

Depending on what you are avoiding, choosing the appropriate type of cuisine makes a big difference; for example, if you eat in a Thai, Japanese or Chinese restaurant, it is relatively easy to avoid dairy and wheat products or meat. Indian restaurants also offer many meat-free alternatives.

If you are entertaining yourself, our recipes and menus will give you plenty of good options. Also, the cookbook *Food GLorious Food* provides a wide selection of recipes from around the world, all low GL. You can use these when you are entertaining and create delicious menus free from the foods you are avoiding – and the chances are your guests won't even notice.

Alcohol is a hard one to avoid when the peer pressure is on, however. A Virgin Mary (spicy tomato juice) is an alcohol-free, low-GL drink that you can get in any bar, although sometimes it is easier – if you have an insistent host – to accept a small glass of wine and either not drink it, or drink it very slowly avoiding top ups. Alternatively, just stick to water. Remember, Rome wasn't built in a day, and the odd deviation from your 'perfect' plan is not the end of the world.

Tips to improve your relationship with food

- Improve your relationship with food by identifying those foods with which you have an emotional charge and then eating small amounts to 'densitise' yourself.
- Notice which foods you use to binge on or eat in excess, or which foods you seem to crave, or eat, on a daily basis, and break the habit.
- Expand your repertoire of foods and dishes.
- Take time for preparing meals, and eating with your family and friends.
- When eating out, choose the style of cuisine that's going to give you the healthiest options.
- Follow your chosen diet six days out of seven, and don't be too hard on yourself when you make the odd deviation.
- Notice what circumstances make you deviate from your perfect diet, and think of alternative ways of dealing with these situations.

10: Eat soul food

We take food, like life, for granted but both are a great blessing. We are made from food. Your skin is new in 21 days, your inner skin – the digestive tract membrane – is new in four days, and even your bones rebuild, made directly from what you put in your mouth. We depend on oxygen from the air; hydrogen and oxygen from water; hydrogen, oxygen and carbon from food (making up carbohydrate and also fat), and nitrogen from the protein in food, plus eight essential vitamins and 18 essential minerals from the earth the plants grow in, as well and hundreds of other plant-based nutrients. We are literally composed of the elements, as well as sunlight, the element of fire. Our internal fire, created by our cell's metabolic processes, gives us not only warmth but also life.

In our 100% Health Survey of the top health scorers, 88 per cent said that they consider spiritual factors were important for health, whereas 81 per cent said they considered themselves spiritual, and 83 per cent said that having a connection with nature was important. Recognising that your incredible body, and ability to sense the wonders of the world, is only possible due to nature providing us with food is part of that spiritual connection. Food is a direct part of nature, as we are and being aware of this makes us appreciate it more. It also makes it taste better.

Expressing gratitude

Fundamental to all religions is the act of grace: expressing gratitude for the food you are about to take in. But you don't have to be religious, or have a belief in God, to be grateful that you are part of this chain of creation, having the food you need to be alive, and the choice and the means to be healthy and to satisfy your senses. Millions of people in the world do not.

The simple act of being aware that the food you are about to receive becomes an essential part of you will help to remind you not to abuse your body with low-quality and toxic food eaten for an immediate sense of pleasure. In fact, all the pleasures you enjoy – whether they be great tastes, stunning views, or the inspiration of art, literature and music, the exhilaration from sex and the buzz you get from energetic sports and exercise, as well as the joy of learning new things – only happen for as long as your body and mind are working well. Your mind, body and senses only function optimally throughout your life if you eat the right foods and take care of yourself.

With this awareness you can choose to express gratitude internally for your food and its gift of keeping you healthy and strong.

Conscious eating

Recently, I went fishing off the coast of Africa and caught a yellow-fin tuna. This creature fought hard to stay alive, using incredible strength. It is a magnificent fish with incredible colours and a streamline design, full of muscle. It made me think about how there is a cycle of life: the tuna's life is sacrificed to support my life, and that of my family and friends. I hate to waste any part of an animal whose life, that elusive and wonderful thing, is sacrificed to support my own. I abhor the way we have thought of animals as just a food factory, and created inhumane and unnatural ways of rearing animals with disregard for their evolutionary heritage. I am also too aware of how we have plundered the oceans with massive trawlers, over-fishing with complete disregard to the food chain, resulting in the elimination of certain species.

Many of the commercial methods that have been introduced to produce cheap food have created food that is nothing like as healthy as it was in the past. A chicken in the 1970s had, on average, 9g (¼oz) of fat. Today, a chicken has, on average, 22g (1oz) of fat. This increase in fat is the result of the bird not having an active life and being fed too much carbohydrate with the intention of fattening it up quickly to make more money for the producer. The same thing happens to us: inactivity and too much carbohydrate makes us fat and unhealthy.

When you buy animal produce, it is worth checking that it the animal is truly a healthy one, reared in humane conditions, not least because your health depends upon it.

The same is true with vegetables. If you grow your own, which is highly rewarding, you can do so without using chemicals, but instead cultivate good, organic soil that will yield crops of nutritious vegetables. The flavour and experience of eating home-grown or organic foods surpasses the bland taste of most mass-produced vegetables. Furthermore, if you were to analyse home-grown or organic versus mass-produced vegetables you would find that those grown without chemicals have a greater nutrient content. So, it is worth spending a little extra to choose good-quality vegetables, both for your health and your enjoyment.

Eat local, seasonal produce

Plants progressively lose their nutrients the longer the time passes between when they were picked and when they are eaten. It is also ecologically unsound to transport food from one side of the world to the other. So, for both of these reasons, it is good to be aware of where the food you eat is grown, and to support local farmers and food growers. Farmers' markets are appearing in many more towns today, providing local produce in season, which is often organic. I eat seasonal foods as often as possible, and I also freeze berries, for example, to eat in the winter months. Freezing super-fresh foods retains most of the nutrients.

Of course, it is beneficial to our health that we have access to some foods when they are out of season, but it is better to choose produce from close to home rather than the other side of the world whenever you can.

How you eat makes a difference

If you eat while watching television, it is possible to become unconscious about what you are eating, disregarding its tastes and textures. Also, if you are watching something designed to increase your adrenalin level that, in turn, switches off your digestion. If you gulp food down in a hurry to get on with whatever job you consider is most important next, you will also be losing out on the experience of eating. Eating then becomes simply an act of rapid refuelling, like a Grand Prix racing car. In contrast, eating with awareness make your meals a pleasurable experience. Some of the happiest communities in the world take their food and meal times seriously, stopping to make a meal and sharing it in good company.

When you eat with awareness you are also more likely to chew your food more thoroughly, which helps to break it down. So, if you find yourself eating unconsciously, a good exercise is to simply put your fork down between mouthfuls. Leave at least 30 minutes between the main course and a dessert, because it takes time for your system to register that it is full. In the Indian tradition you are recommended to fill your stomach half with food and a quarter with water. Digestion is perceived of as the internal fire and, if you fill yourself up too much, you will put out the fire and suffer indigestion. It is good to experiment with eating only until you are just satisfied, and not stuffed.

These simple principles will make food a more fulfilling experience, nourishing both your body and your soul.

Tips for eating soul food

- Express gratitude for the food you are about to eat.
- Choose animal produce from healthy animals, reared humanly and in line with their evolutionary design.
- Choose organic vegetables and fruits.
- Eat as much local produce and seasonal food as you can, freezing foods when in season for the winter.
- Don't waste food.
- Chew your food well and take time to eat it; enjoy eating in good company.

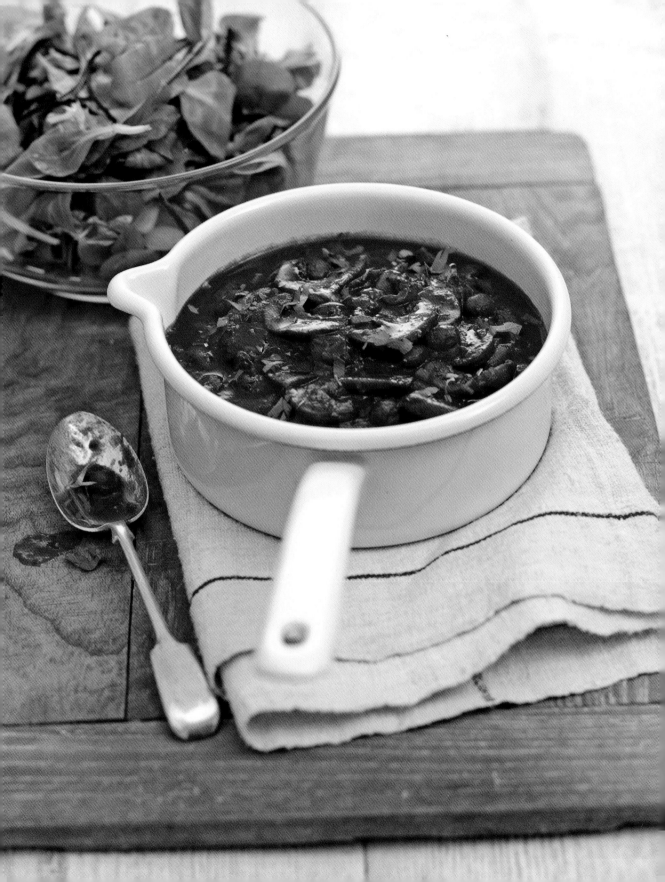

PART TWO

THE RECIPES

By Fiona McDonald Joyce

General guidance on the recipes

I HOPE THAT YOU FIND these recipes useful. It is always hard to change your eating habits, so if you are new to the concept of healthy eating I would like to think that there are enough tempting dishes and ideas in this section to inspire you and to ensure that you enjoy your meals while you try to improve your health. If you are a long-standing follower of Patrick's healthy-eating principles and are familiar with our previous books, I have tried to bring all sorts of refreshing ideas to these pages to ensure that there are plenty of new recipes for everyone. Before you start cooking, the following information may be useful.

Healthy oils and flavourings

When you're preparing food that tastes good to eat as well as being healthy, you need to think carefully about which oils, salt and sweetening are best to use. These recommendations will enhance the flavour of your meals and increase their nutritional value.

Cooking oil

I recommend frying with stable oils such as coconut oil or virgin rapeseed oil, or mild/medium olive oil. These oils are relatively heat resistant, thereby limiting the formation of harmful free radicals. I do not advise that you cook with extra virgin olive oil, because not only is it expensive but also less heat resistant, which means that the heat generated by cooking damages its taste and nutritional value.

Coconut oil can be found in good health-food stores or bought online (see Resources). There are two types: extra virgin, unrefined coconut oil, which is highest in the beneficial lauric acid, and normal, non-virgin coconut oil. The extra virgin oil does have a fairly strong flavour so some people prefer the cheaper non-virgin variety, but it is a matter of personal taste – and budget. Coconut oil is an excellent choice in Asian dishes and dishes which have a full flavour, as it does have a certain distinctive taste that may not always be appropriate. If you want a milder flavoured oil, rapeseed oil is an excellent choice. There are a number of British farms producing first-class extra virgin rapeseed oil, which is rich in both flavour and nutrients and relatively stable when heated.

Salt

Although salt has a place in every kitchen, as far as I am concerned, I would advise caution over quantity and quality of the salt. Avoid heavily processed table salts in preference of unrefined sea and rock salts. These are not only fuller in flavour so that you need to use less but they are also naturally rich in valuable trace minerals such as potassium and magnesium. I prefer to use these rather than the 'low salt' products, as they are a more natural product and the flavour is better.

Xylitol

You will notice that I use xylitol instead of sugar in sweet recipes. This naturally occurring sugar substitute is found in many fruits and vegetables and has the same sweetness as sugar, but you would have to eat nine spoonfuls of xylitol for it to have the same effect on your blood sugar levels as just one spoonful of sugar. This makes it ideal for dieters, diabetics and those following a low-GL diet. Plus, xylitol is naturally antibacterial, preventing bacteria from adhering to teeth and so helping to avoid tooth decay – hence you will find it as an ingredient in many dental products. Although it is not a panacea, and Patrick and I still recommend that you limit sweet foods to the occasional treat, it does mean that you can enjoy favourite foods and drinks without having to add standard sugar. You can find xylitol in most good supermarkets or buy it online (see Resources for more information). You use exactly the same amount of xylitol as you would do standard sugar. If you prefer to use ordinary sugar you will find I have included it as an option in the recipes, although please note that the GL scores given in the recipes are for xylitol not sugar (which would increase the GL score).

About the Cook's Notes

Each recipe contains Cook's Notes which set out the allergy suitability of that particular dish. Please note that this information refers to the ingredients in the recipe itself, not any additional serving suggestions, which should also be taken into consideration if you do have any food allergies.

The Cook's Notes also highlight the following as appropriate:

• Useful preparation and ingredient tips
• V indicates that the recipe is suitable for vegetarians
• Can be prepared in advance
• Suitable for freezing

At-a-glance health scores

Within the Cook's Notes you will find various symbols to denote the recipe's glycemic load (GL) and how much it contributes to your recommended intake of ORAC foods, essential fats and methylation-helping B vitamins (these are discussed in Part One). Here's a guide to what the symbols tell you:

• **ORAC** Our menus and recipes are designed to achieve at least 6,000 ORACs a day (see page 35). As pointed out in Part One, we have assigned the following symbol to denote 1,000 ORACs. Whichever recipes you choose, make sure you get six a day. Also, when you freewheel and create your own menus, if you do choose multicoloured ingredients, covering all the main colours in a day, the chances are you'll achieve the golden 6,000 ORACs (or) guideline.

• **Omega-3 fats** The recipes have also been devised to make it easy to achieve your recommended intake of omega-3 fats (see page 39). Any recipe that contains omega-3 is denoted with a Ω. Your goal, for optimal health, is to achieve three Ω a day. One serving of oily fish gives you $\Omega\,\Omega\,\Omega$, while a serving of white fish gives you $\Omega\,\Omega$ and a tablespoon of chia or flax seeds or sesame seeds, or a small handful of walnuts gives you Ω. Our menus are designed to give you $\Omega\,\Omega\,\Omega$ a day. The best vegetarian sources of omega-3 are chia seeds and flax seeds, followed by hemp, pumpkin seeds and walnuts.

- **B vitamins** To make sure you get a good amount of B vitamins to aid methylation (see page 30), each recipe has been rated on a scale of one to three, using the symbol $\boxed{B}$. One $\boxed{B}$ is scored if a dish contains vegetables, nut or seeds, which are good sources of B vitamins, including B_6. Similarly one $\boxed{B}$ is scored if a dish contains fish, meat, eggs or milk, which all provide vitamin B_{12}. $\boxed{B}\boxed{B}$ is scored if a dish contains beans and pulses, which are particularly rich in folate. If a dish contains two types of vegetable and eggs for example, then it scores $\boxed{B}\boxed{B}\boxed{B}$. You want to achieve $\boxed{B}\boxed{B}\boxed{B}$ every day. So, if you have one recipe with '$\boxed{B}$' and another with '$\boxed{B}\boxed{B}$', you've done it. If you want to achieve this easily at home, eat seven servings of fruit and vegetables a day, with plenty of methylation-boosting green vegetables and citrus fruits, have a small handful of raw nuts or seeds per day and a portion of beans or lentils most days. The daily menus outlined on page 76 achieve this.

Please note that although we have done our best to make the scores in this book as accurate as possible, not all foods have reliable GL or ORAC scores available. In these instances we have had to make a calculated estimate. Also, there are variations in scores according to different sources, and while we have used the same sources throughout in order to minimise inconsistencies, please be aware that GL scores of certain foods may vary depending on which source you look at. Our scores are intended to be a guide only.

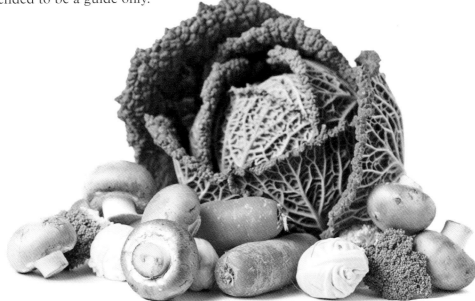

Cooking methods

In keeping with Patrick's recommendation to consume plenty of raw or lightly cooked food, I try to focus on cooking techniques that preserve as many of the ingredients' nutrients as possible. This means plenty of dishes involving steaming, steam-frying or sautéing, and poaching, while avoiding or very much limiting high-temperature cooking methods like deep frying and high-temperature roasting, which can produce harmful free radicals when oil and fats are damaged by excessive heat. Chargrilling and barbecuing also raise health concerns, as such high-temperature cooking produces a group of compounds known as heterocyclic amines or HCAs – potentially carcinogenic chemicals that are formed as a result of the action of heat on amino acids (the building blocks of protein) during the cooking process. Although HCAs can form on many types of food, it seems that it is meat, with its high protein content, combined with a high cooking temperature, that is the most susceptible. If you want to find ways around this problem, consider a gas-fired barbecue, as the temperature can be more readily controlled. Cutting your meat more thinly before cooking will also help it to cook more quickly and therefore limit the opportunity for HCAs to form. Interestingly, evidence has suggested that certain marinades can have an impact on HCA levels; honey-based ones raise HCA levels while garlic, turmeric and teriyaki dressings seem to inhibit HCA formation.

Cooking pans

If you like to use non-stick pans, invest in one of the safer brands that do not release toxic fumes upon reaching certain temperatures, or contain perfluorooctanoic acid (PFOA), a chemical linked to a host of serious health problems. Even the more expensive pans, if given the standard non-stick coating, will do this. The only two such brands of non-stick cookware that I know of that avoid harmful 'off gassing' are Scan Pan and Green Pan, both of which are available in the UK and which I use and recommend. You can find details for both in Resources. A cheaper solution is simply to use stainless steel cookware, although it is not non-stick of course, so you will need to cook with more oil to prevent sticking. I do not advise cooking with pure aluminium pans, because if they come into contact with an acidic food or liquid, they can leach harmful aluminium into your food.

Fresh v. frozen and canned food

If you don't have time to shop for fresh produce as regularly as you would like, or you are on a tight budget, frozen vegetables and fruit, such as berries, have much to recommend them. Keep bags of peas and mixed berries in the freezer. Canned food is also very convenient and canned beans and pulses make it much quicker and easier to prepare meals containing these nutritious ingredients. Avoid cans lined with plastic though, as this could be a source of BPA (bisphenol-A), a hormone disruptor, leaching in to your food.

Steam-frying

The great advantage of steam-frying is that the lower temperature of steaming doesn't destroy nutrients in the way that frying does, and you use only a small amount of oil, if that. Use a shallow pan or a deep frying pan with a thick base and a lid that seals well. Add 1 tsp–1 tbsp of rapeseed or olive oil, butter or coconut oil to the pan, warm it, add the ingredients and sauté. After 2 minutes or so, add 2 tbsp of liquid – this can be water, vegetable stock, soy sauce or a little watered-down sauce that you'll use for the dish – and clamp the lid on. Steam the ingredients until the vegetables are al dente. You can also steam-fry without oil by first adding 2 tbsp of liquid, such as water or stock, to the pan. Once it boils, immediately add some vegetables, then 'sauté' rapidly for 1–2 minutes, turn up the heat, add 1–2 tbsp more of the liquid and clamp the lid on tightly. After 1 minute, add the remaining ingredients. Turn the heat down after 2 minutes and steam in this way until the vegetables are al dente. You can always add more liquid at any time if your pan boils dry.

Menu plans

TO MAKE LIFE EASY, I have included a plan of one week's meals for you, which you can either follow to the letter or simply use as a guide to show you how you might combine different dishes to meet the dietary goals set out in Part One. For the purposes of giving as many different menu permutations as possible, I have suggested new dishes for each meal, but of course if you are preparing meals at home, you could use leftovers for subsequent meals to save time. You might also not have time to prepare lunch each day, so if you are working and want to grab a sandwich or a salad, bear in mind the guidelines given below and in Part One and choose wholemeal bread, a salad, or a bowl of soup or half a jacket potato, for example, and include some sort of protein, such as tuna, chicken, prawns or tofu, as well as vegetables or fruit in some form.

The menu plan on pages 76–77 adheres to the weight-loss requirements of GL eating, so dieters need not worry, and anyone else can simply increase the portion size of any accompaniments such as rice or potatoes (see the portion guide on page 81), or include a pudding, if you like. I have also relaxed the meals over the weekend to include some puddings, while still fitting in with Patrick's guidelines. These guidelines can also be easily followed when planning your own meals.

Menu planning guidelines

Here is a recap of the main goals, which are achieved in the menu plan and which you are advised to try to meet when planning your own meals:

1 Have three meals a day and two snacks. If you wish to lose weight, aim for 10GLs per main meal and 5GLs per snack. If you do not need to lose weight, you can relax this to 15GLs per main meal and 7.5GLs per snack. Patrick also allows an additional 5GLs per day for drinks, making a total of 45GLs for weight loss and 65GLs for weight maintenance.
2 Always combine protein and carbohydrate foods in a meal, to help slow the energy release for better blood sugar balance.

3 Eat multicoloured foods regularly, ideally choosing something yellow, orange, red, green and purple every day.

4 Combine meals to give you 🥕🥕🥕🥕🥕🥕, to ensure you are eating your 6,000 ORACs recommended daily intake.

5 Aim to have at least three servings of oily fish a week, preferably unfried, and four or more servings of fish in total (including white fish) a week.

6 Try a limit red meat to two servings a week or three if one of these is lean game such as venison.

7 Eat some omega-3-rich raw seeds or nuts every day – such as a tablespoon of chia or flax seeds, or a small handful of walnuts or pumpkin seeds. You could have a small handful of raw nuts or seeds, perhaps ground on cereal, added to soups or as a snack with some fruit. If you are a strict vegetarian or vegan you'll need double this amount.

8 Have at least six free-range or organic eggs a week, preferably from chickens fed on omega-3-rich feed.

9 Eat foods rich in methylation-supporting B vitamins, to give you your B B B quota per day:
- Aim for seven servings of fruit and vegetables a day; for example, fruit with breakfast and two fruit snacks, plus two servings of vegetables with each main meal.
- Eat plenty of green vegetables.
- Have a serving of beans or lentils most days. This could be by using beans and pulses in a main meal or simply having a snack of hummus and crudités or oatcakes.

Main Meals

In the recipe section you will find a whole range of low-GL main meal choices, from quick and simple soups and salads for lunch, to main course fish, vegetarian and hearty meat dishes, along with suggested accompaniments. They are rich in vegetables, herbs and spices to provide flavour and nutrients and, as with the menu plans, as long as you watch the size of any accompaniments that you choose to serve alongside the dishes, the vast majority will stay within the 10GL threshold for a meal (see the score per dish for an exact guide). They also provide adequate protein to help keep blood sugar levels in balance, and indeed the meat, fish and eggs are also rich in B vitamins which boost methylation, while the fish section includes a range of oily fish to help you to achieve your recommended weekly omega-3 intake.

Snacks

As Patrick explained in Part One, you can enjoy a morning and afternoon snack when eating according to low-GL principles as long as you make sure that each stays within the 5-GL limit (or 7.5 if you don't need to lose weight). Some simple snacks that do just that include fresh fruit, such as an apple, a couple of plums, or a bowl of berries, ideally eaten with a small handful of unsalted, unroasted nuts or pumpkin seeds. These serve to provide some protein to slow the rate of sugar release from the fruit as well as helping to meet your daily recommended intake of a tablespoon of nuts or seeds. Other ideas include avocado, olives, hummus spread on oatcakes, or crudités with a dip such as guacamole or hummus. Dried fruit is a popular snacking choice but it is also a concentrated source of fruit sugars, so limit it to a small handful or avoid it entirely in favour of fresh fruit.

If you want to make up a snack mix to keep in your bag, in your desk at work or in the larder ready for an instant energy boost, try making your own trail mix. Combine nuts and seeds, such as hazelnuts, walnuts, Brazil nuts, almonds and pumpkin seeds, perhaps with a few goji berries to add a burst of sweetness and juiciness (as well as including a considerable amount of vitamins and minerals). If you want to enliven it somewhat, add cacao (raw, unprocessed chocolate) nibs, and perhaps a dusting of cinnamon. Keep the mix in a glass jar or bottle and shake to combine the ingredients evenly.

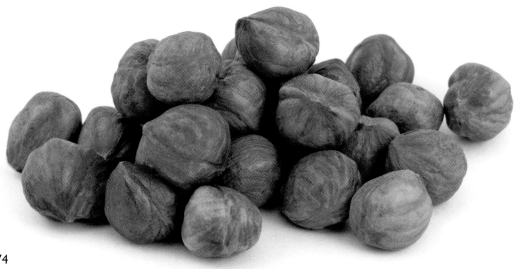

Drinks giving 5 GLs

Drink	5 GLS
Tomato juice	600ml (20fl oz/1 pint)
Carrot juice	1 small glass
Grapefruit juice, unsweetened	1 small glass
Cherry Active concentrate	1 small glass, diluted 50:50 with water
Apple juice, unsweetened	1 small glass, diluted 50:50 with water
Orange juice, unsweetened	1 small glass, diluted 50:50 with water; or juice of one orange
Pineapple juice	half a small glass, diluted 50:50 with water
Cranberry juice drink	half a small glass, diluted 50:50 with water
Grape juice	2.5cm (1in) of liquid!

Note 1 small glass = 175ml (6fl oz)

Drinks

In his low-GL diet, Patrick allows for 5GLs per day for drinks. Be aware that it is not only sweetened squashes and soft drinks that will raise the GL of a drink, the natural sugar content of pure fruit juices and smoothies will do the same. The chart above shows you what you could drink and how much, for 5GLs.

Milk contains some milk sugar, so if you drink lots of milky teas and coffees, then that will also use up your 5-GL quota. Healthier, zero-GL alternatives include water, of course, and herbal teas.

As for alcohol, Patrick advises that a regular, although not daily, drink (say four times a week) does not present a big health issue and that small quantities of 'dry' drinks such as dry wine, champagne, dry lager or spirits such as whisky are not a concern in terms of GL. It is the mixers like cola and orange juice that are more of an issue for blood sugar levels. Of course, the resveratrol content of red wine also makes it an excellent high-ORAC choice!

Sample menu plan

Here is your first week's – or your sample week's – menus:

	Monday	Tuesday	Wednesday
Breakfast	Poached Eggs on Soda Bread (page 94), plus optional piece of fruit	Blueberry Yoghurt Sundae (page 83), plus optional slice rye toast or Seeded Spelt Bread (page 170), topped with nut butter or yeast extract	Porridge with Almonds and Goji Berries (page 89)
Lunch	Broccoli Soup (page 102), plus slice Seeded Spelt Bread (page 170) or wholemeal bread, or 2 oatcakes	Peruvian Quinoa Salad (page 116) with a green salad	Smoked Salmon-stuffed Avocado (page 118) with a mixed salad
Dinner	Thai Chicken and Cashew Stir-fry (page 125) with brown basmati rice and Stir-fried Choi Sum in Oyster Sauce (page 174)	Baked Trout with Lemon and Almonds (page 137), with Herby Puy Lentils (page 169) or new potatoes and steamed Tenderstem broccoli or salad	Sweet Potato and Chickpea Stew (page 156) with salad or Braised Kale with Almonds (page 176)
Snacks	Apple and a small handful of raw nuts or seeds Crudités with hummus	2 apricots or plums and a small handful of raw nuts or seeds Crudités with guacamole	Pear and a handful of raw nuts or seeds Small pot of live natural yoghurt (or soya yoghurt) and berries

Thursday	Friday	Saturday	Sunday
Hot Smoked Trout with Scrambled Eggs and Watercress (page 84), plus optional slice of wholemeal toast	Apple and Hazelnut Granola (page 93) plus optional stewed fruit	Cinnamon Oat Pancakes (page 92) with berry compote	Salmon and Asparagus Omelette (page 86), plus optional slice wholemeal toast, Chia Loaf (page 168) or Seeded Spelt Bread (page 170), with nut butter or yeast extract
Beetroot and Borlotti Bean Soup (page 105)	Bacon, Avocado and Tomato Mix (page 114) plus slice Chia Loaf (page 168) or Seeded Spelt Bread (page 170) or wholemeal bread, and spinach, rocket and watercress salad	Olive, Pine Nut and Feta Salad (page 120) with green leaf salad, followed by Pineapple, Pomegranate and Mint Fruit Salad (page 182)	Venison and Chocolate Stew (page 132) with Celeriac and Potato Rösti (page 159) and Savoy Cabbage with Chestnuts (page 175)
Cumin-spiced Meatballs (page 134) with Herby Puy Lentils (page 169) or wholemeal spaghetti and salad	Sun-dried Tomato Pesto with Cannellini Beans (page 160) (or replace beans with wholemeal pasta) and Peperonata (page 173)	Thai Lamb Red Curry (page 128) with brown basmati rice or quinoa, followed by Chocolate Espresso Mousse (page 181)	Barley and Vegetable Broth (page 99) followed by Greek Yoghurt and Cherry Pots (page 185)
Berries and a small handful raw nuts or seeds Crudités with cottage cheese or hummus	Pear and a handful of raw nuts or seeds Small pot or bowl of live natural yoghurt (or soya yoghurt) with berries	Crudités and hummus Apple and a handful of raw nuts or seeds	Crudités with guacamole Pear and a handful of raw nuts or seeds

Table of dishes and scores

The chart below lists all the recipes, with their GL, ORAC, essential fat and vitamin B content per serving as well as page numbers to help you find them. This is intended to be an easy reference guide to help you plan your own meals and meet the guidelines in Part One.

Health scores guide

Dish	GL	ORAC	Essential fats	B vitamins	Page
Breakfasts					
Blueberry Yoghurt Sundae	3	🥕🥕🥕🥕🥕	-	BB	83
Hot Smoked Trout with Scrambled Eggs and Watercress	0	-	ΩΩΩ	BBB	84
Kippers with Wilted Spinach	0	-	ΩΩΩ	BB	85
Salmon and Asparagus Omelette	1	-	ΩΩΩ	BBB	86
Wild Mushrooms on Toast	10	-	-	B	88
Porridge with Almonds and Goji Berries	3	🥕	-	BB	89
Chia Pancakes with Pear Compote	6	🥕🥕🥕	Ω	BB	90
Cinnamon Oat Pancakes	7	🥕🥕	-	B	92
Apple and Hazelnut Granola	4	🥕🥕	-	BB	93
Poached Eggs on Soda Bread	6	-	-	B	94
Spiced Honey Drizzle	3	🥕🥕🥕🥕	-	-	95
Bircher Muesli	6	🥕🥕🥕🥕🥕🥕🥕	Ω	BBB	96
Spiced Apple with Yoghurt	5	🥕🥕🥕🥕🥕	Ω	BB	97
Soups					
Barley and Vegetable Broth	5	🥕🥕	-	BBB	99
Curried Pumpkin Soup	8	🥕🥕🥕🥕	-	BBB	100
Broccoli Soup	6	🥕🥕	-	BB	102
Oliver's Celeriac and Watercress Soup	7	🥕	-	BBB	103
Beetroot and Borlotti Bean Soup	6	🥕🥕	-	BBB	105
Raw Red Pepper and Tomato Soup	2	-	-	BBB	106
Haddock Chowder	7	🥕	ΩΩ	BBB	107
Coconut Milk and Mushroom Broth	3	🥕 (estimate)	-	B	108
Salads					
Wild Rice, Artichoke and Aduki Bean Salad	10	🥕	Ω	BBB	111
Butternut Squash and Tenderstem Salad	3	🥕🥕🥕🥕	Ω	BBB	113

Dish	Score	Carrots	Omega	B	Page
Bacon, Avocado and Tomato Mix	3	✂ ✂	-	ⒷⒷⒷ	114
Pearl Barley and Bean Salad	8	-	-	ⒷⒷⒷ	115
Peruvian Quinoa Salad	8	✂ ✂	Ω	ⒷⒷⒷ	116
Smoked Salmon-stuffed Avocado	3	✂ ✂	Ω Ω	ⒷⒷ	118
Super-greens Salad	2	✂ ✂ ✂ ✂ ✂	Ω	ⒷⒷⒷ	119
Olive, Pine Nut and Feta Salad	3	✂ ✂ ✂ ✂	-	ⒷⒷⒷ	120
Main meals – meat					
Chicken and Puy Lentil One-pot Stew	7	✂ ✂ ✂ ✂ ✂ ✂	-	ⒷⒷⒷ	123
Thai Chicken and Cashew Stir-fry	5	✂	-	ⒷⒷⒷ	125
Slow-cooked Pork with Winter Vegetables	10	✂	-	ⒷⒷⒷ	126
Shepherd's Pie with Sweet Potato Topping	9	✂ ✂ ✂	-	ⒷⒷⒷ	127
Thai Lamb Red Curry	5	-	-	ⒷⒷⒷ	128
Simple Beef, Onion and Mushroom Stew	4	✂ ✂ ✂ ✂ ✂	-	ⒷⒷⒷ	130
Pumpkin and Bacon One Pot	8	✂ ✂ ✂	-	ⒷⒷⒷ	131
Venison and Chocolate Stew	2	✂ ✂ ✂ ✂	-	ⒷⒷⒷ	132
Cumin-spiced Meatballs	1	✂ ✂ ✂ ✂ ✂	-	Ⓑ	134
Quinoa Jambalaya	4	-	-	ⒷⒷⒷ	135
Main meals – fish					
Baked Trout with Lemon and Almonds	0	-	Ω Ω	ⒷⒷ	137
Thai Salmon Noodle Bowl	8	-	Ω Ω Ω	Ⓑ	139
Steamed Trout with Ginger	0	-	Ω Ω Ω	ⒷⒷⒷ	140
Patrick's Super-healthy Kedgeree	8	✂ ✂ ✂ ✂	Ω Ω	ⒷⒷⒷ	141
Steamed Salmon with Soy and Garlic Spring Greens	1	-	Ω Ω Ω	ⒷⒷ	142
Smoked Paprika-spiced Tilapia with Tenderstem	3	✂ ✂	Ω Ω	ⒷⒷ	143
Garlic Chilli Prawns	1	✂	-	ⒷⒷ	144
Pan-fried Pollock and Sweet Potato Chips	7	-	Ω Ω	ⒷⒷ	146
Fish Medley in a White Sauce	7	-	Ω Ω Ω	ⒷⒷ	147

Recipe					Page
Monkfish Wrapped in Parma Ham	0	-	Ω Ω	B	148
Omelette with Smoked Haddock, Parmesan and Chives	0	-	Ω Ω	B B	150
Main meals – vegetarian					
Vegetable Steam-fry	1	🥕	-	B B B	152
Lentil Dahl	6	🥕 🥕 🥕	-	B B B	153
Bean and Mushroom Bolognese	7	🥕 🥕 🥕 🥕 🥕	-	B B B	154
Sweet Potato and Chickpea Stew	8	🥕	-	B B B	156
Quinoa Pilaf with Red Pepper and Pumpkin Seeds	5	-	Ω	B B B	157
Celeriac and Artichoke Frittata	4	-	-	B B B	159
Sun-dried Tomato Pesto with Cannellini Beans	2	-	-	B B B	160
Vegetable Quinoa Curry	9	🥕 🥕	Ω	B B B	161
Baked Sweet Potato Topped with Goat's Cheese and Sun-dried Tomatoes	7	🥕	-	B B	162
Peppers Stuffed with Wild Rice	9	🥕 🥕	Ω	B B	164
Cauliflower, Chickpea and Egg Curry	9	🥕 🥕 🥕	-	B B B	165
Tofu Noodle Stir-fry	15	-	Ω	B B B	166
Accompaniments					
Chia Loaf	7	🥕	Ω	B B B	168
Herby Puy Lentils	7	🥕	Ω	B B B	169
Seeded Spelt Bread	5	-	Ω	B B B	170
Celeriac and Potato Rösti	7	-	-	B B	172
Peperonata	1	🥕 🥕 🥕 🥕 🥕	-	B B B	173
Stir-fried Choi Sum in Oyster Sauce	1	🥕 🥕	-	B	174
Savoy Cabbage with Chestnuts	1	-	-	B B	175
Braised Kale with Almonds	1	🥕	-	B B	176
Puddings and sweet treats					
Chocolate Crunchies	8	🥕 🥕 🥕	Ω	B B	179
Coconut Cups	2	-	-	-	180
Chocolate Espresso Mousse	4	🥕 🥕 🥕 🥕 🥕 🥕	-	B	181
Pineapple, Pomegranate and Mint Fruit Salad	4	🥕 🥕 🥕	-	-	182
Greek Yoghurt and Cherry Pots	7	🥕 🥕 🥕 🥕 🥕 🥕 🥕 🥕	Ω	B B	185
Blueberry Jellies	4	🥕 🥕 🥕	-	-	186
Pineapple Sorbet	5	🥕	-	-	187

Accompaniment serving sizes

When it comes to knowing how much rice, pasta or potatoes to serve with your meals, you can vary the portion according to whether you want to stick to the 45GLs per day weight-loss limit or relax this a bit to 65 GLs to maintain weight. Here is a handy reference guide to show you roughly how much of each of the healthiest carbohydrate choices you could eat.

Portion guide

Food	7 GLs approximate serving (for weight loss)	10 GLs approximate serving (for weight maintenance)
Brown basmati rice (raw)	40g (1½oz)	60g (2oz)
Wholemeal pasta (dried)	40g (1½oz)	55g (2oz)
Quinoa (raw)	65g (2¼oz)	95g (3¼oz) (NB very large serving)
Baked potato/sweet potato	½ small	1 small
Boiled baby new potatoes	75g (2¾oz) (about 3)	125g (4½oz) (about 4)
Beans, pulses (approximate value; different types can vary)	½ × 410g can	¾ × 410g can
Rough milled oatcakes	4	5–6
Rye bread (e.g. pumpernickel or sourdough)	1 slice is 10 GLs	1 slice
Wholemeal wheat bread	1 slice is 10 GLs	1 slice

BREAKFASTS

A GOOD BREAKFAST should set you up for the day without leaving you feeling
bloated and heavy before you even start work, or light-headed and lethargic from
unbalanced blood sugar levels. The key to getting your energy levels in check for the
rest of the day is to choose a low-GL option, which will not only avoid a blood sugar
spike but has also been shown to 'calibrate' your body's blood sugar response to
subsequent meals; so start as you mean to go on by choosing a source of slow-releasing
energy. These recipes provide plenty of protein to help slow down the rate of the release
of energy from food, to help keep blood sugar levels in balance. There are plenty of
whole-grain options like the Apple and Hazelnut Granola on page 93 and fruit-based
dishes like the Blueberry Yoghurt Sundae shown below. I have also included three
different types of egg dishes, to help you achieve Patrick's recommendation of eating six
or more eggs per week.

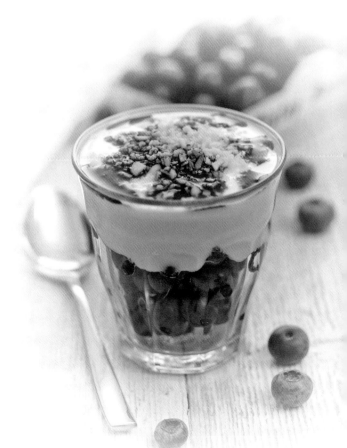

BLUEBERRY YOGHURT SUNDAE

This breakfast is bursting with colour and natural sweetness from the antioxidant-laden blueberries and Cherry Active cherry juice. This is a great choice for dieters, as eating blueberries daily appears to improve insulin sensitivity. If you have digestive problems, try sheep's or goat's yoghurt, as they tend to be better tolerated, or use soya yoghurt to make this entirely dairy-free.

Serves 1

3 heaped tbsp blueberries

3 heaped tbsp live natural yoghurt or sheep's, goat's or soya yoghurt

4 tsp ground chia seeds, or other seeds or flaked almonds

2 squirts of Cherry Active (see Resources), or blueberry juice

1 Put the blueberries into a wide glass or a dessert bowl.

2 Spoon the yoghurt over the berries, then scatter the seeds or almonds over the top.

3 Finish by drizzling the Cherry Active or blueberry juice over the top.

Cook's Notes

Allergy suitability: gluten/wheat/yeast/dairy free (if using soya yoghurt)

V • Can be made in advance

Health scores per serving: GL 3 • 🥕🥕🥕🥕🥕 • B B

HOT SMOKED TROUT WITH SCRAMBLED EGGS AND WATERCRESS

This is a '10 Secrets' winner, combining omega-3 fats from the oily fish with B vitamin-rich eggs and dark green leafy vegetables. It makes an excellent weekend breakfast for when you have a bit more time to treat yourself. It tastes particularly good served on hot buttered rye toast, or one of the whole-grain bread recipes in this book.

Serves 1

knob of butter or coconut oil

2 free-range or organic eggs

pinch of sea salt

1 hot smoked trout fillet

small handful watercress, roughly chopped

freshly ground black pepper

wedge of lemon, to serve

1 Melt the butter or oil in a small pan over a gentle heat and crack the eggs into the pan. Add the salt and stir with a wooden spoon to mix. Put the toast on at this point.

2 Slowly stir the eggs with a wooden spoon, scraping along the base of the pan as they cook to keep them moving and help stop them sticking. Remove from the heat as soon as the eggs are almost set but still a little runny/moist, as they will carry on cooking in the pan.

3 Spoon the eggs on to a plate, then put the trout fillet on top, sprinkle with black pepper, then scatter the watercress over the top. Serve immediately with a wedge of lemon on the side.

Cook's Notes

Allergy suitability: gluten/wheat/dairy/yeast free (depending on butter or oil)

Health scores per serving: GL 0 • $\Omega\,\Omega\,\Omega$ • $\boxed{\text{B}}\,\boxed{\text{B}}\,\boxed{\text{B}}$

KIPPERS WITH WILTED SPINACH

'Proper' kippers (not the boil-in-the bag, lurid dyed kippers from the supermarket shelf) are well worth hunting out from the fishmonger and paying a little extra for. As an oily fish, they provide omega-3 essential fats as well as protein. This is perfect served with whole-grain toast such as rye bread.

Serves 1

1 undyed, naturally smoked kipper, filleted
handful of baby leaf spinach
knob of butter or extra virgin olive oil (optional)

freshly ground black pepper
wedge of lemon, to serve

1 Grill the kipper for about 5 minutes or until heated through.

2 Meanwhile, throw the spinach into a small pan over moderate heat and let it wilt for 1 minute or so. Add a small knob of butter or a drizzle of oil, if you like.

3 Serve the kipper with the spinach and lemon wedge and sprinkle with plenty of black pepper.

Cook's Notes

Allergy suitability: wheat/dairy free (if not using butter)
Health scores per serving: GL 0 • $\Omega\,\Omega\,\Omega$ • $\boxed{B}\,\boxed{B}$

SALMON AND ASPARAGUS OMELETTE

This dish ticks a lot of boxes, with the oily fish providing omega-3, the egg providing a hefty dose of B vitamins for methylation and the green vegetables adding fibre and vitamins. You can take this recipe and vary it according to taste or what you have in the fridge – try wilted spinach and sun-dried tomatoes, or perhaps stir-fried shiitake mushrooms as an omelette filling.

Serves 1

3 free-range or organic eggs
pinch of sea salt
50g (2oz) fine asparagus spears, trimmed
knob of butter or coconut oil

1 heaped tbsp diced smoked salmon (more if you like)
freshly ground black pepper
wedge of lemon, to serve

1 Beat the eggs and salt together in a bowl.

2 Put the asparagus on to steam for about 5 minutes or until al dente – take care to take it off the heat as soon as it is cooked. While this is cooking, make the omelette.

3 Heat a small frying pan over a medium heat, add the butter or oil and move it about the pan to coat the base and sides, then pour in the eggs. As the omelette starts to set, repeatedly run the back of a fork across the base of the pan to lift up some of the mixture and let the uncooked egg spill underneath and cook.

4 When the base has coloured and set, put the asparagus over half the omelette and top with the smoked salmon. Sprinkle with black pepper, then carefully fold in half and leave for 30 seconds or so to cook the middle before easing it out of the pan and onto a plate. Serve immediately, with a wedge of lemon.

Cook's Notes
Allergy suitability: gluten/wheat/dairy/yeast free (if using oil not butter)
Health scores per serving: GL 1 • $\Omega\Omega\Omega$ • BBB

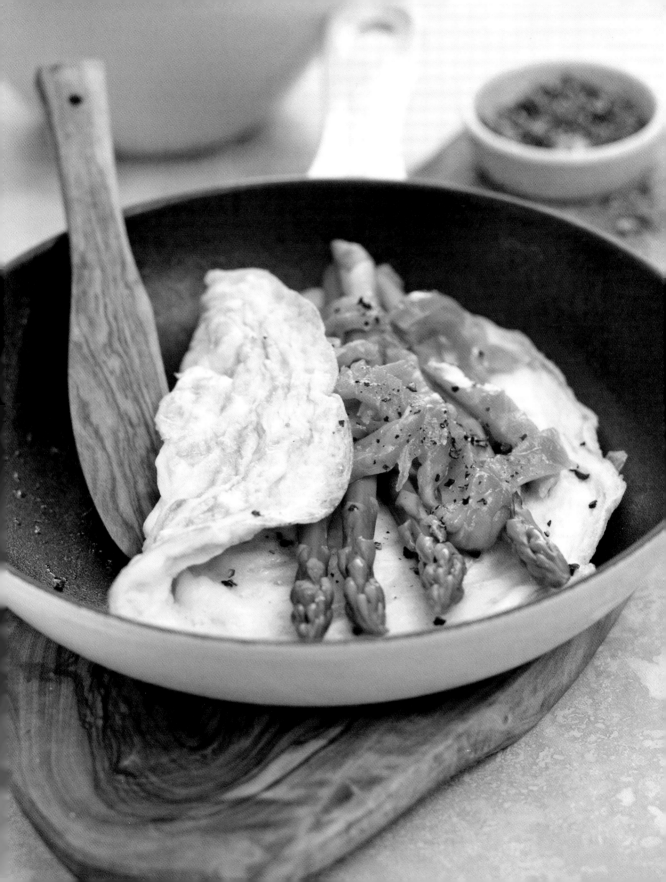

WILD MUSHROOMS ON TOAST

Strongly flavoured wild mushrooms are quite delicious served simply, on hot buttered toast. I suggest using rye bread, as it is particularly good at helping to control blood sugar response. You might like to add some lightly wilted spinach to increase your green leafy veg quota. Perhaps have a boiled egg, or some yoghurt or a handful of nuts or pumpkin seeds in addition to this dish to complete your breakfast, to boost the protein content. This recipe serves two, as wild mushrooms are normally an occasional treat when you can get hold of them, so it makes a nice weekend breakfast or brunch to share. However, if you are just treating yourself, simply halve the quantities.

Serves 2

25g (1oz) butter, plus a little for spreading, or coconut oil

75g (3oz) wild mushrooms (or white, button or chestnut mushrooms), brushed or wiped

2 slices whole-grain toast, wheat-free if preferred

freshly ground black pepper

a little sea or rock salt

flat-leaf parsley sprig or finely chopped chives

1 Add the butter or oil to a hot frying pan then, when melted, add the mushrooms and fry over a moderate heat until soft and coloured. Make the toast while the mushrooms are cooking.

2 Season to taste and drain (mushrooms contain a lot of water).

3 Butter the toast and spoon the mushrooms on top. Garnish with a sprig of flat-leaf parsley or the chives and serve.

Cook's Notes

Allergy suitability: wheat/yeast free (if using wheat and/or yeast-free bread like sourdough or some rye breads) • V

Health scores per serving: GL 10 • Ⓑ

PORRIDGE WITH ALMONDS AND GOJI BERRIES

Many people steer clear of nuts for fear of their high fat content, but research suggests that the high fibre content of almonds, for example, actively limits absorption of fat from the nuts. The protein content also makes nuts very low GL. If you cannot find goji berries, try chopped dried apricots instead, and try to buy organic or unsulphured dried fruit in order to avoid the use of the preservative sulphur dioxide, a potential allergen.

Serves 1

4 tbsp porridge oats

water or milk/non-dairy milk, or a 50:50 blend, in a ratio of 2 parts liquid to 1 part oats

2 tsp–1 tbsp goji berries

1 tbsp flaked almonds

1 Put the oats in a small pan. Add double the amount of water, milk or a blend of both.

2 Bring to a gentle simmer and allow to bubble and thicken for a few minutes, until the oats have swollen.

3 Pour into a bowl, then sprinkle with goji berries and almonds before serving.

Cook's Notes

Allergy suitability: wheat/dairy/yeast free (depending on milk) • V

Health scores per serving: GL 3 • 🔪 • B B

CHIA PANCAKES WITH PEAR COMPOTE

These little pancakes make an interesting alternative to a traditional pancake or drop scone, replacing processed white flour with milled oats and chia seeds. They are just as moreish but wheat free, low GL and high in antioxidants. If you cannot get hold of chia seeds (see Resources), substitute ground almonds or flax seeds, or simply use double the quantity of oats instead. This recipe makes enough for four people, but the pancakes keep well for a couple of days in the fridge or can be frozen.

Serves 4 (makes 8 pancakes)

For the pear compote

2 large pears, cored and diced

dash of water

1 tsp ground mixed spice or cinnamon, or to taste

xylitol (or brown sugar), to taste (optional)

45g (1½oz) oats

45g (1½oz) milled chia seeds

35g (1¼oz) xylitol (or sugar)

1 free-range or organic egg

225ml (8fl oz) milk or non-dairy milk

virgin rapeseed oil for frying

1 To make the pear compote, first stew your pears by putting them in a small pan with a tiny dash of water and the spice. Bring to a simmer, cover and leave to cook for 5 minutes, or until just softened. Taste and add more spice if you like. You could sweeten the mixture with xylitol or brown sugar if you feel it needs it. Set aside, with the lid on, while you make the pancakes.

2 Grind the oats with the chia into as fine a flour as you can. If your food processor leaves the mixture coarse, try a hand blender to achieve a smoother finish.

3 Mix the xylitol into the flour.

4 Whisk the egg and milk together and stir into the flour mixture to form a smooth batter. The chia absorbs liquid, so it will thicken more than a standard pancake batter.

5 Heat 1–2 tbsp oil in a large frying pan, then spoon in tablespoonfuls of the batter, spreading each out into a rough circle and taking care not to let them touch. Do this in batches and cook each pancake for 1–2 minutes per side, or until golden and firm. Press down in the pan to flatten the cooked pancakes. Cover with a tea towel to keep warm while you work. Serve with the stewed fruit.

Cook's Notes

Allergy suitability: wheat/dairy/yeast free (if using non-dairy milk) • V • Can be frozen

Health scores per serving: GL 6 • 🥕🥕🥕 • Ω • BB

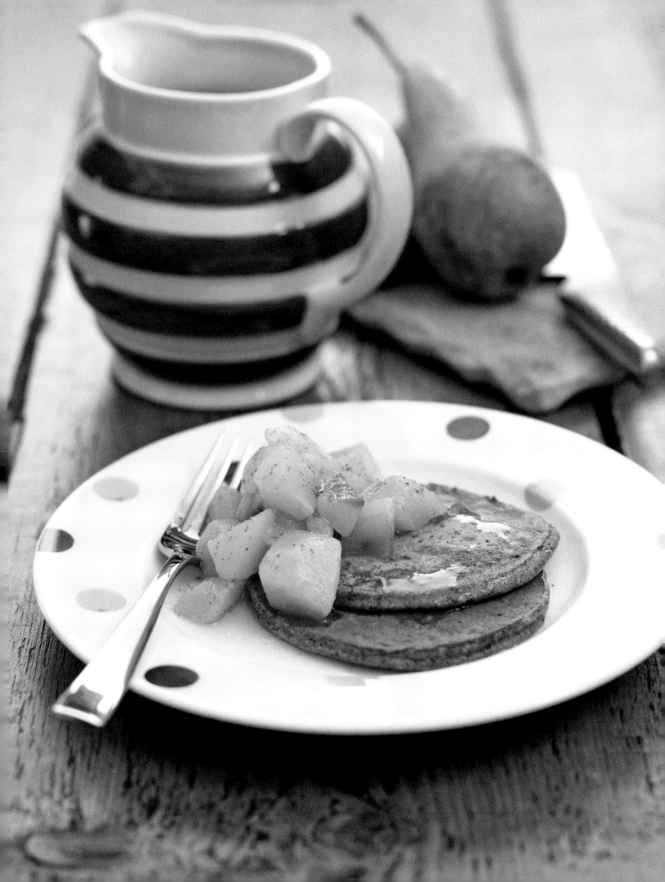

CINNAMON OAT PANCAKES

This recipe, as in the Chia Pancakes on page 90, uses ground oats instead of refined wheat flour. This makes these pancakes easier to digest, as oats do not contain gliadin, the type of gluten found in wheat that is particularly hard to digest. Plus, this is of course rich in the valuable vitamins, minerals and fibre found in whole grains. Simply scrummy with a squeeze of lemon juice and a sprinkling of xylitol instead of sugar, or with stewed fruit. If you have any leftovers, they can be stored in the fridge for a few days and reheated.

Serves 6–8

115g (4oz) whole oat flakes, finely ground to
    form a flour (using a food processor)
2–3 tsp cinnamon
35g (1¼oz) xylitol (or sugar)
1 free-range or organic egg

270ml (9fl oz) milk or non-dairy milk
virgin rapeseed oil for frying
lemon juice, xylitol (or caster sugar) or stewed
    fruit, to serve

1 Mix the oat flour, cinnamon and xylitol or sugar in a bowl. Taste the batter before cooking, if you like, to get your preferred level of cinnamon.

2 Lightly beat the egg and milk together, then stir into the dried ingredients to form a runny mixture. If the mixture is not particularly smooth it may be that your blender isn't powerful enough to grind the oats to a fine flour, so blend the mixture quickly using a hand-held blender to make it as smooth as possible. The mixture may thicken up if left for a while, but you can loosen it by adding a little more milk.

3 Heat a tablespoon of oil in a large frying pan and tip the pan to coat the base, then pour tablespoonfuls of the pancake mixture into the pan (without touching each other). Fry for 1 minute or so on each side, or until firm and golden brown (do this in batches so as not to crowd the pan). Put the pancakes onto a warmed plate as they cook, and cover with a tea towel to keep warm. Serve the pancakes warm with lemon juice and xylitol or with stewed fruit.

Cook's Notes
Allergy suitability: wheat/dairy/yeast free (if using non-dairy milk) • V • Can be frozen
Health scores per serving when serving 8: GL 7 • 🥕🥕 • B

APPLE AND HAZELNUT GRANOLA

Research has shown that it is best to eat hazelnuts with their skin still on, as that is where much of their antioxidant content can be found. I have also included wheat germ in this recipe because it is an incredibly rich source of folic acid, to help with methylation. The dried apple lends natural sweetness, while the oats and xylitol instead of sugar make this much lower GL than most granolas. Enjoy served with fresh berries and live natural yoghurt.

Serves 4

2 tbsp coconut oil or mild or medium (not extra virgin) olive oil or virgin rapeseed oil

150g (5½oz) whole oat flakes, or a blend of oat and barley flakes

3 tbsp hazelnut butter

3 tbsp whole (skin on) hazelnuts, chopped

1 tbsp milled chia seeds (see Resources) or milled flax

1 tbsp wheat germ, or seeds if you prefer it to be wheat-free

2 tbsp finely chopped dried apple slices

1 tbsp xylitol (or brown sugar)

2 tsp ground mixed spice

1 Gently melt the oil in a frying pan, then add the oats and stir to coat evenly. Cook for 1 minute or so to start to crispen slightly.

2 Mix in the hazelnut butter as best as you can to coat evenly.

3 Stir in the remaining ingredients. Taste and adjust the flavour by adding more sweetness or spice as preferred. Leave to cool, then store in an airtight container for instant breakfasts.

Cook's Notes

Allergy suitability: wheat/dairy/yeast free (if no wheat germ) • V • Can be made in advance
Health scores per serving: GL 4 • 🥕🥕 • B B

POACHED EGGS ON SODA BREAD

Poaching is one of the healthiest ways of serving eggs, as the gentle cooking method preserves more of the valuable phospholipids and B vitamins. This soda bread recipe is delicious and dead easy, but if you want a quick cheat, try the Rankin brown soda bread from supermarkets, which is an excellent shop-bought alternative. Serve with cherry tomatoes, if you like.

For the soda bread (Makes 2 loaves, each serving about 8 slices – eat one and freeze the other)

450g (1lb) wholemeal flour (not strong bread flour)

½ tsp sea salt

2 tsp baking powder

1 tsp bicarbonate of soda

2 tsp soft brown sugar (don't use xylitol or another kind of sugar, as the loaf will lose its flavour and be too sweet)

300ml (10fl oz/½ pint) milk and water mixed

1 tbsp plain natural yoghurt

For the poached eggs. Serves 1

2 organic or free-range eggs

freshly ground black pepper

pinch of sea or rock salt

1 Preheat the oven to 220°C/425°F/Gas 7 and grease a baking tray. To make the soda bread, put the flour, salt, baking powder and bicarbonate of soda in a food processor and blend for 10 seconds to combine.

2 Dissolve the sugar in the milk and water mixture, then stir in the yoghurt and add to the dry ingredients. Process for another 10 seconds, then scrape the sides and blitz for a further 5 seconds to thoroughly blend the mixture. If the mixture is not quite firm you can gradually add another tablespoon or two of flour to the mixture, keeping the motor running as you do so, until the dough leaves the sides of the bowl clean. (Alternatively, to make it without a food processor, put the dry ingredients, except for the sugar, in a large bowl and stir in the wet ingredients with the dissolved sugar until well combined.)

3 Take the dough out of the bowl and shape it into two round, fairly flat loaves (like large buns). Put the loaves on the baking tray, leaving as much space as possible between them, and cover each one with a large, ovenproof bowl, leaving enough space for the loaves to rise. Bake for 30 minutes.

4 Remove the bowls and return the loaves to the oven to bake for a further 10 minutes, then allow to cool for 10–15 minutes.

5 To poach the egg, pour freshly boiled water into a saute pan over a very gentle heat so that there is the merest hint of bubbles and movement. Put your bread in to toast at this point, then crack the eggs into the pan carefully and allow to gently poach in the water for about 3 minutes or until the tops no longer look transparent.

6 Butter your bread if it is warm from the oven, or toast to reheat. Remove the cooked poached egg from the pan and allow to drain, then season and serve on the bread.

Cook's Notes
Allergy suitability: yeast free • V
Health scores per serving: GL 6 per slice soda bread • B̲

SPICED HONEY DRIZZLE

This has become a daily staple in our household. Turmeric is an incredibly powerful anti-inflammatory spice used in India for medicinal purposes. Cinnamon is not only a good source of ORACs but also helps the body to cope with sugar, making it the perfect partner to the honey. Drizzle this mixture over live natural yoghurt or porridge, or spread it on toast.

Serves 1
¾ tsp ground turmeric
½ tsp ground cinnamon
1 tsp fresh lemon juice

about 1 tsp very good quality honey, such as Manuka (see Cook's Notes)
1 tsp hot water

1 Mix the turmeric and cinnamon together in a very small bowl.

2 Add the lemon juice, honey and hot water.

3 Stir well to fully combine the mixture and produce a smooth, runny paste.

4 Taste and add a little more honey if you want to reduce the strength of the spices. You can adjust the quantity or proportions of spices, lemon juice and honey according to taste.

Cook's Notes
Organic forest honey is another alternative to Manuka. Look for one that is cold pressed and with no sugar or antibiotics used.
This is particularly good as a tonic when you are fighting off a cough, cold or sore throat.
Allergy suitability: gluten/wheat/dairy/yeast free• V • Can be made in advance
Health scores per serving: GL 3 • 🥕🥕🥕🥕 per serving

BIRCHER MUESLI

A meltingly soft, slightly chewy mixture of fruity goodness that is quite delicious. Wheat germ is an excellent source of folic acid, to help with methylation. I think this is sweet enough on its own, thanks to the dried apple and the bursts of blueberry, but if you prefer, you could add ½ tsp xylitol, honey or brown sugar. You could also add a drizzle of Cherry Active (concentrated cherry juice – see Resources), to really send the ORAC score through the roof.

Serves 1

4 tbsp oat flakes

1 tbsp wheat germ, or ground almonds if you prefer it wheat-free

1 tbsp ground almonds, or flaked for a coarser texture

1 tbsp pumpkin seeds, or another type of seed or nut

1 tsp ground cinnamon, or to taste

10g (¼oz), or about a heaped tbsp, finely chopped dried apple rings

3 tbsp frozen or fresh blueberries

150ml (5fl oz/¼ pint) milk or non-dairy milk

1 Put the oats in a bowl. Mix in the wheat germ, almonds, seeds and cinnamon.

2 Add the apples and blueberries and pour in the milk. Stir to coat everything, then cover.

3 Chill in the fridge for an hour to let the oats swell and soften, or make the night before, ready for breakfast the next morning. You can always add more sweetness, cinnamon, berries or milk to change the flavour or consistency if you like.

Cook's Notes

Allergy suitability: wheat/dairy/yeast free (if omitting the wheat germ and using non-dairy milk)

V • Can be made in advance

Health scores per serving: GL 6 • 🥕🥕🥕🥕🥕🥕🥕 • Ω • Ⓑ Ⓑ Ⓑ

SPICED APPLE WITH YOGHURT

A healthier take on a fruit fool that replaces cream with live natural yoghurt to help digestion, and which also includes antioxidant-rich cinnamon and walnuts. This light, simple breakfast could also be enjoyed as a snack between meals. This keeps well in the fridge for five days.

Serves 4

about 775g (1lb 11oz) or 4 medium Bramley (cooking) apples, peeled, cored and roughly chopped
dash of water
about 1 tbsp xylitol (or brown sugar), to taste

about 2 tsp ground cinnamon, or to taste
8 heaped tbsp Greek live natural yoghurt (or soya yoghurt)
4 tbsp walnut pieces, roughly chopped

1 Put the apples in a pan with the water. Bring to the boil, then reduce the heat to a gentle simmer, cover and cook for 8–10 minutes or until the apple is disintegrating.

2 Season to taste with xylitol or sugar and cinnamon.

3 Allow to cool, then stir into the yoghurt.

4 Spoon into four bowls and scatter with walnuts before serving. This keeps well in the fridge.

Cook's Notes

Allergy suitability: gluten/wheat/yeast/dairy free (if using soya yoghurt) • V

Can be made in advance • Suitable for freezing

Health scores per serving: GL 5 • 🥕🥕🥕🥕🥕 • Ω • 𝔹𝔹

SOUPS

SOUPS HAVE BEEN SHOWN to leave you feeling fuller for longer, making them an ideal choice for lunch during a busy working day, or simply if you are trying to control your appetite while on a diet. Some soups can be heavily laden with cream or cheese, or flour thickeners; these recipes are hearty and filling, but lighter on fat and fillers. Read through the selection and you will also notice the sheer range of colours, from the vivid green Broccoli Soup on page 102 (surprisingly delicious, so do please give it a go) to the rich orange of the Curried Pumpkin Soup on page 100 and the deep purple of the Beetroot and Borlotti Bean Soup on page 105. This makes them a great way to eat a rainbow of different colours for optimal antioxidant intake. If you want to have a slice of bread with your bowl of soup, just check the GL score in the Cook's Notes for each recipe, and if you are trying to keep your GL points per meal to within 10 to lose weight, choose a lighter option such as the Raw Red Pepper and Tomato Soup on page 106. Do look at the Accompaniments on page 168 and 170 as well, where you will find some recipes for home-made breads that feature whole grains and which are likely to have a lower GL than most shop-bought versions.

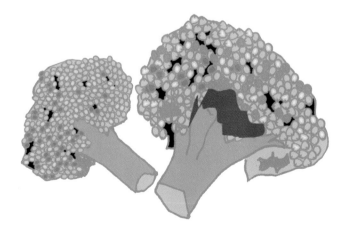

BARLEY AND VEGETABLE BROTH

This is a very hearty, filling soup, and yet the GL is very low, thanks to the high vegetable content and the lentils and barley. In addition, research over many years has shown that barley seems to help to keep cholesterol levels in check.

Serves 4

2 tbsp mild or medium (not extra virgin) olive oil, or virgin rapeseed oil or coconut oil, or 40g (1½oz) butter

2 carrots, diced

1 leek, thinly sliced

3 celery sticks, finely sliced

1 thyme sprig

115g (4oz) pearl barley, rinsed and drained

50g (2oz) red lentils, rinsed and drained

1.2 litres (2 pints) vegetable or chicken stock

2 tbsp finely chopped flat-leaf parsley

2 tbsp finely chopped baby spinach, watercress or rocket

sea or rock salt

freshly ground black pepper

1 Heat the oil or butter in a pan and add the carrots, leek and celery. Sauté for about 5 minutes so that the vegetables start to soften.

2 Stir in the thyme, barley, lentils and stock, bring to a simmer, then cover and cook for about 45 minutes, or until the pearl barley is soft to the bite and the vegetables are very tender.

3 Remove the thyme stalk, stir in the chopped parsley and greens, and season to taste.

Cook's Notes

Allergy suitability: gluten/wheat/dairy/yeast free (depending on stock, and if using oil not butter)

V (if using vegetable stock) • Can be made in advance

Health scores per serving: GL 5 • 🥕🥕 • B B B

CURRIED PUMPKIN SOUP

Including spices like cumin and curry powder is a great way to boost the ORAC content of a dish effortlessly, as they are real star performers in the antioxidant stakes. This warming, brightly coloured soup is an excellent choice if you are trying to fight off a bug or you have a sore throat.

Serves 4

1 tbsp mild or medium (not extra virgin) olive oil, virgin rapeseed oil or coconut oil

1 large or 2 small red onions, chopped

2 garlic cloves, crushed

2 tsp mild or medium curry powder

900g (2lb) pumpkin or butternut squash, cut into cubes

1 large carrot, chopped

800ml (28fl oz) hot chicken or vegetable stock

a little sea or rock salt

freshly ground black pepper

4 tbsp finely chopped or blended (with a little extra virgin olive or rapeseed oil) baby spinach leaves

1 Heat the oil in a large frying pan, add the onions, garlic and curry powder and sauté for 1 minute. Add the pumpkin or squash cubes and carrot, and sauté for a further 10 minutes to pick up some colour.

2 Transfer the mixture to a large pan or stock pot and add the stock. Bring to the boil then reduce the heat, cover and simmer for 15 minutes.

3 Blend until smooth then season to taste.

4 Ladle the soup into bowls then place a spoonful of the chopped or blended spinach in the middle of each bowl.

Cook's Notes

Allergy suitability: gluten/wheat/dairy/yeast free (depending on stock used) • V (depending on stock)

Can be made in advance • Suitable for freezing

Health scores per serving: GL 8 • 🥕🥕🥕🥕 • B B B

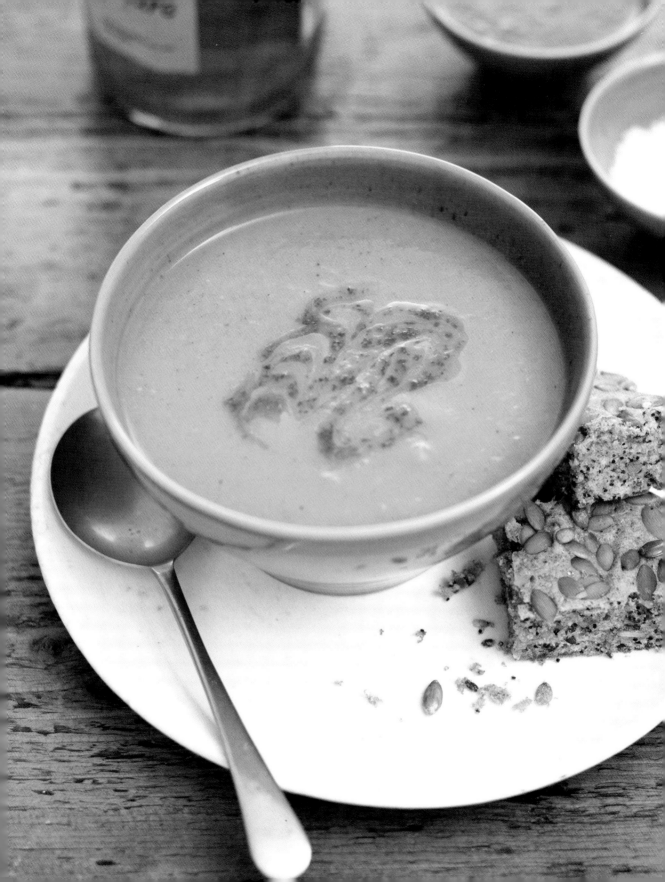

BROCCOLI SOUP

This has become a weekly favourite in our household and, brilliantly, it is just as popular with my two-year-old son as it is with the adults. This is much better tasting than its simple ingredients would suggest, so do give it a try. It is a quick and easy way to increase your intake of methylation-boosting greens. This recipe serves just two because cooking it fresh each time gives you maximum benefit from the vivid green goodness of the broccoli, although you can double up if you want to have some leftover for next time or are serving four people.

Serves 2

1 tbsp mild or medium (not extra virgin) olive oil, virgin rapeseed oil or coconut oil
2 garlic cloves, crushed
500ml (18fl oz) hot vegetable stock (see Cook's Notes)

400g (14oz) broccoli, cut into florets
100ml (3½fl oz) milk or non-dairy milk such as Kara coconut milk or oat, rice or soya milk
freshly ground black pepper

1 Heat the oil in a large pan, add the garlic and gently sauté for 1 minute or so, taking care not to let it burn.

2 Add the stock and the broccoli, and bring to the boil.

3 Reduce the heat, cover and simmer for 10 minutes, or until the broccoli is tender.

4 Add the milk and plenty of black pepper, then blend with a stick blender until smooth. Adjust the seasoning if necessary.

Cook's Notes

Non-vegetarians could use chicken stock instead of vegetable stock for added flavour.
Allergy suitability: gluten/wheat/dairy/yeast free (depending on stock and milk used)
V • Can be made in advance • Suitable for freezing
Health scores per serving: GL 6 • 🥕🥕 • ⒷⒷ

OLIVER'S CELERIAC AND WATERCRESS SOUP

So called because my toddler son 'helped' me to make this recipe the first time, which, judging from his enthusiasm, is the start of a love of cooking. Celeriac is much lower in starch than potato, making it a good low-GL choice. Top with a small slice of soda bread with grilled goat's cheese slices on top for a more impressive lunch or starter.

Serves 3–4

25g (1oz) butter (or dairy-free spread or coconut oil)

½ tbsp olive or rapeseed oil

2 leeks, sliced

½ medium celeriac, diced

750ml (1¼ pints) hot vegetable stock

115g (4oz) watercress

freshly ground black pepper

a little sea or rock salt, to taste

1 Melt the butter with the oil in a large pan, then add the leeks, cover and sauté for about 10 minutes to soften.

2 Add the celeriac and stock, cover and bring to the boil, then reduce the heat to simmer for about 15 minutes, to allow the celeriac to soften.

3 Add the watercress and blend until smooth. If you are making this ahead of time, you could blend after step 2 and freeze or chill, adding the watercress before serving to maximise its goodness and colour.

4 Season to taste.

Cook's Notes

Allergy suitability: gluten/wheat/dairy/yeast free (depending on stock used) • V

Can be made in advance • Suitable for freezing

Health scores per serving (when serving 4): • GL 7 • 🥕 • B B B

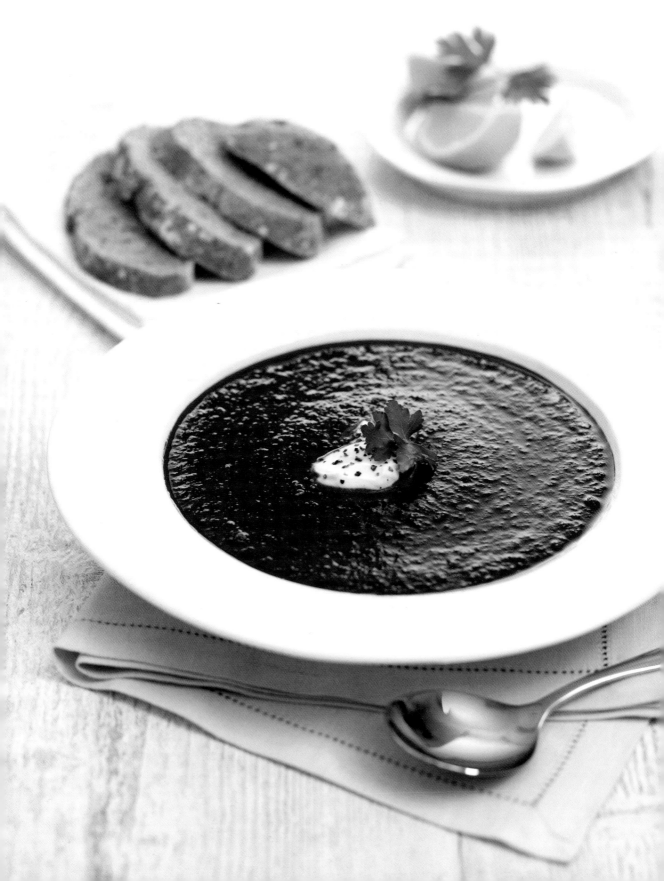

BEETROOT AND BORLOTTI BEAN SOUP

A bright red, thick and filling soup, which could be served warm or cold. You could save time by using cooked beetroot (without vinegar), and blend this up as soon as the onions have cooked. Borlotti beans have a good, almost smoky flavour and are, of course, a source of B vitamins to aid methylation.

Serves 4

1 tbsp mild or medium (not extra virgin) olive oil or virgin rapeseed oil

1 large or 2 small red onions, roughly chopped

2 garlic cloves, crushed

700g (1½ lb) raw beetroot, peeled and diced

400g can borlotti beans, rinsed and drained

800ml (28fl oz) hot vegetable stock

large handful fresh flat-leaf parsley, stalks removed

large handful of fresh mint leaves

juice of 1 lemon

freshly ground black pepper

sea or rock salt to taste

4 tbsp live Greek-style natural yoghurt, to serve (optional)

1 Heat the oil in a pan, add the onion and garlic and gently sauté for 3–4 minutes to soften.

2 Add the beetroot, beans and stock. Bring to the boil, cover and simmer for 15–20 minutes or until the beetroot is fairly tender.

3 Add the herbs and lemon juice, and blend until smooth.

4 Season to taste. Pour into bowls and add a dollop of natural yoghurt in the middle of each, if using.

Cook's Notes

Allergy suitability: gluten/wheat/dairy/yeast free (depending on stock used and if not using yoghurt)

V • Can be made in advance • Suitable for freezing

Health scores per serving: GL 6 • 🥕🥕 • Ⓑ Ⓑ Ⓑ

RAW RED PEPPER AND TOMATO SOUP

This soup is similar in concept to a traditional gazpacho, with the addition of peppers and cayenne pepper to add more antioxidants and flavour, as well as avocado, which is an impressive source of carotenoids. The fact that it undergoes no cooking or heating means that it also retains as many nutrients as possible. This serves two, as it is best served fresh, although the quantities can be increased to feed more or provide leftovers.

Serves 2

1 red pepper, stalk, pith and seeds removed
5 ripe tomatoes
½ cucumber
1 garlic clove, crushed
juice of 1 lemon
1 tbsp extra virgin olive oil

2 handfuls fresh flat-leaf parsley, stalks
   removed
pinch cayenne pepper
1 ripe avocado, diced
freshly ground black pepper
a little sea or rock salt

1 Put the pepper, tomatoes, cucumber, garlic, lemon juice, olive oil, parsley and cayenne pepper in a food processor and blend until smooth or fairly smooth.

2 Stir in the diced avocado.

3 Season to taste – you can add more cayenne if you want it to pack more of a punch.

Cook's Notes
Allergy suitability: gluten/wheat/dairy/yeast free • V • Can be made in advance
Health scores per serving: GL 2 • B B B

HADDOCK CHOWDER

I have tried to keep this recipe lighter than a more traditional chowder, by avoiding very high-GL potato in favour of lower-starch celeriac. This recipe is also very nice if you coarsely blend the soup before serving or before adding the fish, to give a thicker and creamier consistency.

Serves 2–3

25g (1oz) butter or dairy-free spread
1½ tbsp olive or rapeseed oil
2 leeks, sliced
½ medium celeriac, finely diced
300ml (10fl oz/½ pint) milk or non-dairy milk
300ml (10fl oz/½ pint) hot vegetable stock

250g (9oz) skinned and boned undyed smoked haddock
small handful of fresh flat-leaf parsley, leaves roughly chopped
freshly ground black pepper
squeeze of fresh lemon juice (optional)

1 Melt the butter with the oil in a large pan, add the leeks, and cover and sauté for about 5 minutes to soften.

2 Add the celeriac, milk and stock, cover and bring to the boil, then reduce the heat to a simmer for about 15 minutes, to allow the celeriac to soften.

3 Add the fish and gently poach for 2 minutes or until it flakes easily.

4 Break the fish into chunks and season with parsley, pepper and a squeeze of lemon. The haddock should provide sufficient saltiness.

Cook's Notes

Allergy suitability: gluten/wheat/dairy/yeast free (depending on milk and stock)
Health scores per serving: (when serving 3) • GL 7 • $\not{f}$ • $\Omega\,\Omega$ • $\boxed{B}\,\boxed{B}\,\boxed{B}$

COCONUT MILK AND MUSHROOM BROTH

This Asian-inspired broth is so full of flavour that it is well worth sourcing the ingredients to make it. It is wonderfully soothing if you are feeling under the weather, and the coconut milk lends a creamy smoothness despite the fact that this recipe is dairy-free. This recipe serves two because it is best made fresh, but by all means increase the quantities to feed more.

Serves 2

700ml (1¼ pints) hot chicken or vegetable stock
200ml (7fl oz) coconut milk
½ tbsp tamari or soy sauce
½ tbsp Thai fish sauce

1–2 tsp Thai tom yum paste
1 tsp xylitol (or palm sugar or demerara sugar)
6 very thin slices galangal or ginger
15g (½oz) mixed dried wild mushrooms
chopped coriander to garnish (optional)

1 Pour the stock into a medium pan and bring to the boil. Add the coconut milk and boil the mixture for about 5 minutes.

2 Lower the heat to a gentle simmer and then add the tamari or soy sauce, fish sauce, tom yum paste, xylitol or sugar, galangal or ginger and the mushrooms. Leave the soup to simmer, uncovered, for a further 20 minutes or so, until the mushrooms have softened.

3 Taste to check the seasoning before serving and sprinkle with coriander if using.

Cook's Notes
Allergy suitability: gluten/wheat/dairy-free (depending on sauces and stock used)
Can be made in advance
Health scores per serving: GL 3 • 🥕 • B

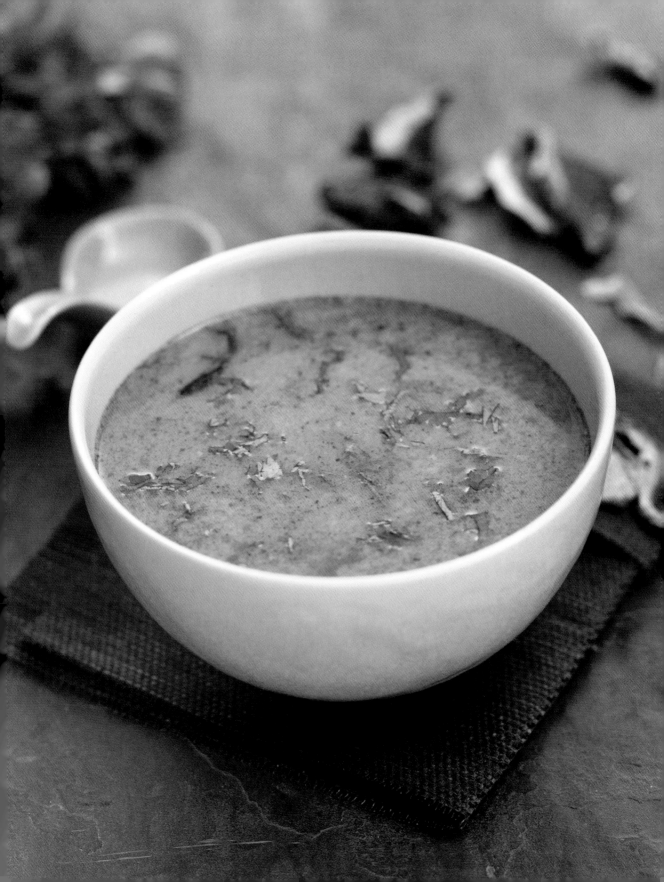

SALADS

A SALAD CAN BE A brilliantly quick meal option, not to mention an extremely healthy one. A salad for lunch is also a great way of making sure that you eat some raw food each day, as advised by Patrick in Part One. Here, I have tried to tempt you with some inventive dishes that make good use of a wealth of different cuisines and ingredients, from the Peruvian Quinoa Salad on page 116 to the more Mediterranean Olive, Pine Nut and Feta Salad on page 120. You will also notice the range of different-coloured ingredients, in a bid to help boost your ORAC score. Brightly coloured plants contain valuable antioxidants, from the anti-inflammatory flavonoids in red onions to the skin-supporting carotenoids in orange-fleshed foods such as butternut squash. A salad can also easily constitute a main meal, as these recipes show, simply by adding more nutritionally dense foods such as nuts or seeds, and starch-based ingredients like squash, beans or quinoa to your bowl of leafy green vegetables.

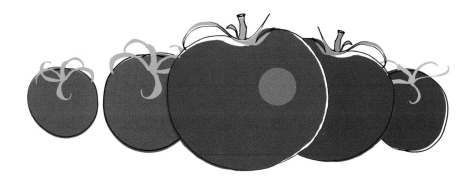

WILD RICE, ARTICHOKE AND ADUKI BEAN SALAD

These small, russet-coloured beans are good source of B vitamins to help methylation, as well as being rich in minerals. Wild rice is not in fact a rice but a grass and is high in protein, making it lower GL than ordinary rice. It takes much longer to cook, but look out for the quick-cook variety.

Serves 4

175g (6oz) wild rice (quick cook if possible), rinsed and drained

400g can aduki beans, rinsed and drained (see Cook's Notes)

4 tbsp pumpkin seeds

about 125g (4½oz) marinated artichoke hearts, drained and chopped

juice of 1 lemon

about 3 tbsp extra virgin olive oil, or to taste

rough handful of flat-leaf parsley, finely chopped

freshly ground black pepper

sea or rock salt, to taste

1 Cook the wild rice according to the pack instructions.

2 When the water has been absorbed, or drained, as required, stir in the aduki beans, pumpkin seeds and artichoke hearts.

3 Squeeze in the lemon juice and add plenty of olive oil. Season to taste, sprinkle with parsley and serve warm or cold.

Cook's Notes

You can use other beans or lentils if you can't find aduki beans.

Allergy suitability: gluten/wheat/dairy/yeast free (depending on ingredients in the marinated artichoke hearts) • V • Can be made in advance

Health scores per serving: GL 10 • 🥕 • Ω • BBB

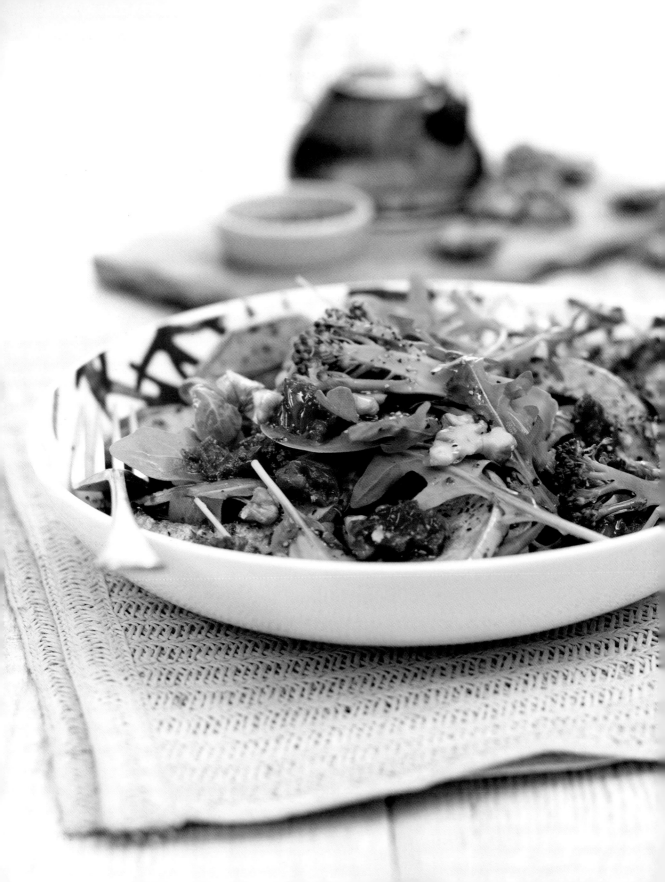

BUTTERNUT SQUASH AND TENDERSTEM BROCCOLI SALAD

The bright colours of this salad are a good clue to its high ORAC content. Tenderstem broccoli is higher in antioxidants than standard broccoli and the orange butternut squash is an excellent source of carotenoids to help skin and eyes. This can be served while the squash is still warm or at room temperature.

Serves 3–4

½ butternut squash, deseeded and chopped into fairly thin slices (no need to peel unless you prefer to)

2 tsp dried oregano

1–2 tbsp mild or medium (not extra virgin) olive oil, or virgin rapeseed oil, for drizzling

200g (7oz) Tenderstem broccoli

about 115g (4oz) mixed leaves, such as rocket, watercress, baby spinach and lamb's lettuce

2 tbsp roughly chopped sun-dried or sunblush tomato pieces in oil, drained

50g (1oz) walnut halves, roughly chopped

vinaigrette salad dressing (optional)

1 Preheat the oven to 220°C/425°F/Gas 7. Toss the squash in the oregano and a little oil to coat, then put on a baking tray. Roast for about 25–30 minutes or until tender, then set aside.

2 Steam the broccoli for about 3 minutes or until just tender, then rinse in cold water to stop it cooking, and dry in a tea towel. Slice into sticks.

3 Put the leaves in a salad bowl, then add the squash and broccoli. Throw in the tomato and walnut pieces, then dress with a vinaigrette.

Cook's Notes

Allergy suitability: gluten/wheat/dairy/yeast free (depending on any marinade oil for the sun-dried tomatoes) • V

Health scores per serving when serving 4: GL 3 • 🥕🥕🥕🥕 • Ω • BBB

BACON, AVOCADO AND TOMATO MIX

Here is a really good salad mixture reminiscent of a BLT, just a bit healthier. By chopping up the bacon and mixing it with salad ingredients, you make a little go a long way. Serve with rocket or other green leaves, and perhaps a slice of the Chia Loaf on page 168. It is also a good sandwich filling in its own right. Don't make this too far in advance because the avocado will discolour. If you do prepare it a few hours ahead, cover and chill, and add the avocado at the last minute.

Serves 3

150g (5½oz) streaky bacon
2 ripe avocados
2 tomatoes, diced
2 spring onions, finely sliced

good pinch sea salt
juice of ¾ lemon
freshly ground black pepper

1 Grill the bacon until crisp. Leave to cool and finely slice.

2 Stone and dice the avocados, then put them into a large bowl.

3 Mix the bacon and remaining ingredients into the bowl and stir to combine. The creaminess of the avocados should start to coat the mixture. Taste and adjust the seasoning as necessary.

Cook's Notes

Allergy suitability: gluten/wheat/dairy/yeast free
Health scores per serving: GL 3 • 🥕🥕 • Ⓑ Ⓑ Ⓑ

PEARL BARLEY AND BEAN SALAD

A very filling mixture that is good served with a simple tomato salad. If you can get hold of pot barley (unrefined barley) so much the better, as the GL score would be lower, but it is hard to find. The combination of beans and grains makes this a balanced source of vegetarian protein, while the beans also make this a good source of nutrients for methylation.

Serves 4

115g (4oz) pearl barley, rinsed and drained
400g can aduki beans, rinsed and drained
1 red onion, very finely sliced
½ small or ¼ large cucumber, finely diced
good handful mint leaves, finely chopped
good handful flat-leaf parsley leaves, finely
   chopped

3 tbsp extra virgin olive oil or rapeseed oil
juice of 1 lemon, or to taste
115g (4oz) feta cheese, crumbled
freshly ground black pepper
 a little sea or rock salt, to taste

1 Put the pearl barley in a pan, cover with cold water and bring to the boil. Drain and rinse with cold water, then return to the pan, re-cover with cold water and bring back to the boil. Reduce the heat to a simmer and cook for 1 hour 15 minutes or until soft to the bite.

2 Drain any excess liquid and set aside to cool.

3 Meanwhile, put the beans, onion, cucumber, mint and parsley in a bowl. Drizzle with oil and lemon juice, carefully fold in the barley and feta, then season to taste with a little salt and plenty of pepper.

Cook's Notes

Allergy suitability: wheat/yeast free • V • Can be made in advance
Health scores per serving: GL 8 • B B B

PERUVIAN QUINOA SALAD

As quinoa originates from the Andes, I thought I should take inspiration from a traditional serving style – a sort of taboulleh with bags of fresh salad herbs and vegetables. Quinoa is a healthier choice than bulghur wheat or couscous as it is gluten-free and very high in protein, as well as minerals like calcium and zinc. I have included pumpkin seeds to further increase the mineral content. Serve with green leaves or on its own.

Serves 4

300g (10½oz) quinoa, well rinsed

1 good handful coriander leaves, finely chopped

2 good handfuls flat-leaf parsley leaves, finely chopped

8 spring onions, finely sliced

1 garlic clove, crushed

4 tbsp pumpkin seeds

half a cucumber, finely diced

200g (7oz) cherry tomatoes, thinly sliced or diced

juice of up to 4 limes, or to taste

good drizzle (about 4 tbsp) cold pressed, virgin rapeseed or olive oil

a little sea or rock salt

freshly ground black pepper

2 ripe avocados, diced

vinagrette salad dressing (optional)

1 Put the quinoa in a large pan, cover with double the amount of water and bring to the boil. Cover and simmer for about 12–13 minutes or until the water is absorbed and the grains are soft and fluffy.

2 Stir the fresh herbs through the quinoa along with the remaining ingredients. Add the avocado just before serving. Taste to check the seasoning. Add the vinaigrette, if using, just before serving.

Cook's Notes

Allergy suitability: gluten/wheat/dairy/yeast free • V • Can be made in advance
Health scores per serving: GL 8 • 🥕🥕 • Ω • 🅱🅱🅱

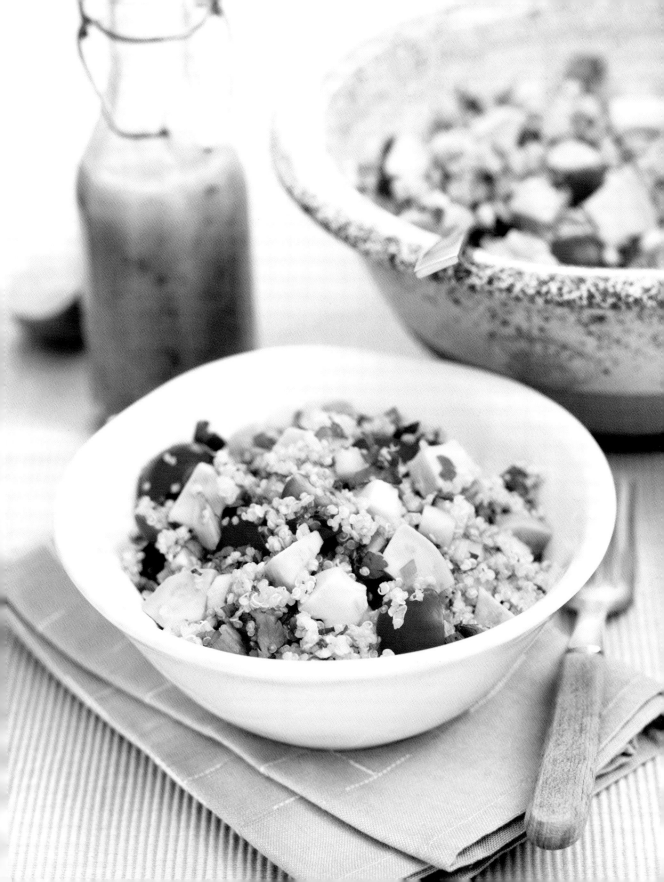

SMOKED SALMON-STUFFED AVOCADO

Avocado is a real wonder food, it is both a rich source of carotenoids and it aids the absorption of two key carotenoids, lycopene and beta-carotene. This is such a simple dish but absolutely delicious if the avocado is ripe. Scrape the darker flesh from the edge of the shell, as this is where the carotenoid concentration is at its highest.

Serves 1

1 ripe avocado

3 tbsp smoked salmon trimmings, or chopped
  smoked salmon strips

freshly ground black pepper

about 2 tsp lemon juice

finely chopped dill, to garnish (optional)

1 Slice the avocado in half lengthways and carefully remove the stone. Scoop out the flesh, taking care not to puncture the skin. Reserve the empty shells.

2 Mash the avocado and stir in the salmon. Season to taste with black pepper and lemon juice.

3 Spoon the avocado mixture back into the shells as neatly as possible. Garnish with a little fresh dill, if you like.

Cook's Notes

Allergy suitability: gluten/wheat/dairy/yeast free • Can be made in advance (best eaten fresh, but this can be kept in the fridge if made a little beforehand)

Health scores per serving: GL 3 • 🥕🥕 • ΩΩ • BB

SUPER-GREENS SALAD

Sprouted beans are a very rich source of nutrients such as B vitamins, and the sprouting process makes the beans more digestible. I have thrown as many nutrient-dense ingredients as possible into this salad, making it a colourful blend of vitamins, fibre and antioxidants. Serve on a bed of dressed mixed leaves such as spinach, watercress, lamb's lettuce and rocket. This salad only serves two as it doesn't keep well as leftovers, but you can easily double the quantities if you have more mouths to feed.

Serves 2

1 tbsp mild or medium (not extra virgin) olive oil, or virgin rapeseed oil

½ red onion, diced

115g (4oz) mixed sprouts (such as Acornbury sprouted aduki beans, chickpeas and lentils), rinsed and drained

1 tbsp walnuts, chopped

6 marinated sun-dried tomatoes, drained and finely chopped

1 tbsp pine nuts

1 tbsp extra virgin olive oil

1 tbsp finely chopped flat-leaf parsley leaves

1 tbsp finely chopped basil leaves

2 tsp dried oregano

2 tbsp lemon juice

1 large, ripe avocado, stoned and diced

freshly ground black pepper

sprinkle of sea or rock salt, to taste

1 Heat the mild oil in a frying pan. Add the onion and mixed sprouts, and stir-fry for about 5 minutes (the sprouts do need cooking).

2 Add the nuts and stir-fry for a further minute or so.

3 Remove from the heat and put into a mixing bowl. Stir in the remaining ingredients, adding the avocado at the end in order not to make the avocado too mushy. Season to taste and serve immediately.

Cook's Notes

Allergy suitability: gluten/wheat/dairy/yeast free (depending on the marinating oil for the sun-dried tomatoes) • V •Can be made in advance

Health scores per serving: GL 2 • 🥕🥕🥕🥕🥕 • Ω • B B B

OLIVE, PINE NUT AND FETA SALAD

Strong Mediterranean flavours and vivid colours make this a perfect summer lunch. It is a high scorer in the ORAC stakes too and feta is a sheep's or goat's milk cheese, making it easier to digest than ordinary cow's milk cheeses. Serve as it is or stuff into a wholemeal pitta bread. The quantities here serve two, as the salad won't last well once the feta has been added, but you can easily double up to feed more people.

Serves 2

50g (2oz) Kalamata olives, halved

25g (1oz) sun-dried tomatoes, chopped

75g (3oz) feta cheese, chopped or crumbled

2 tbsp pine nuts

2 tsp dried oregano

juice of ¼ lemon

freshly ground black pepper

2 small, ripe tomatoes, diced

115g (4oz) mixed leaves, such as rocket, spinach and watercress

1 Mix the olives, sun-dried tomatoes, feta, pine nuts, oregano, lemon juice and pepper together in a bowl.

2 Stir in the fresh tomatoes and the leaves.

3 Taste to check the flavour and adjust if necessary.

Cook's Notes

Allergy suitability: gluten/wheat/yeast free (depending on what the olives are stored in) • V

Can be made in advance

Health scores per serving: GL 3 • 🥕🥕🥕 • B B B

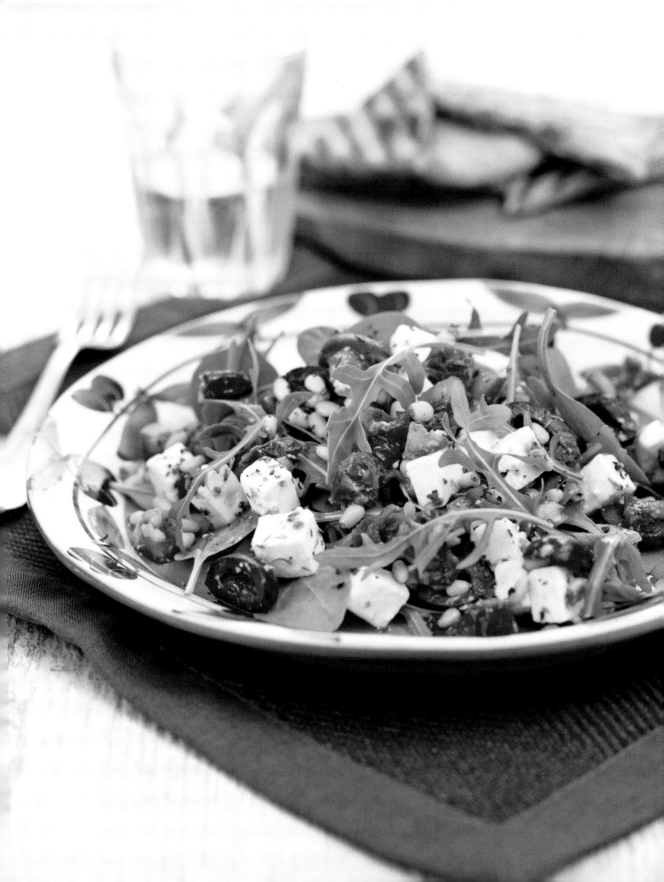

MEAT

I AM A CONFIRMED MEAT EATER, unlike Patrick, but while I wouldn't want to give up the valuable protein and minerals, not to mention taste, of meat, I do recognise that it is sensible to eat meat as part of a balanced diet that is also very rich in plant-based foods. Vegetables, for example, provide the raw materials to help your body produce the digestive enzymes that we need in order to break down foods like meat, and so it is always a good idea to include some sort of vegetable accompaniment, be it a side salad or just some boiled peas, with your meal. These recipes are designed with this in mind, and the plentiful use of vegetables and plant-based starches such as pulses and root vegetables also means that the ratio of meat to vegetables is naturally lowered. The recipes provide a balance of types of meat, from lean poultry to iron-rich red meat and game, to offer different nutritional benefits while also helping you to keep your intake of saturated fat, for example, in balance.

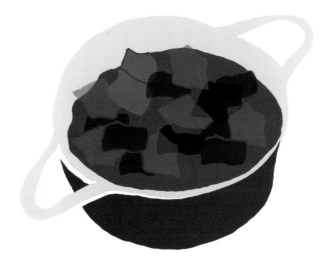

CHICKEN AND PUY LENTIL ONE-POT STEW

Puy lentils are the only type of lentil to hold their shape once cooked, avoiding the mushy consistency that puts many people off these highly nutritious legumes. They also add protein and folic acid, making this a good choice to help with methylation. This hearty stew is a balanced meal on its own, but you could also serve it with some steamed savoy cabbage or spring greens, and the Celeriac and Potato Rösti on page 172, or some mashed sweet potato.

Serves 4

2 tbsp coconut oil or medium or mild (not extra virgin) olive oil or virgin rapeseed oil

16 shallots, peeled and left whole, or 4 large red onions, cut into wedges

4 garlic cloves, crushed

250g (9oz) button mushrooms

4 tsp ground coriander

4 tsp ground cumin

1 tbsp grated or finely chopped fresh root ginger

8 tbsp tomato purée

2 carrots, thinly sliced

2 celery sticks, sliced

1 litre (1¾ pints) hot chicken stock

200g (7oz) dried Puy lentils

4 large chicken thighs, or 8 smaller thigh fillets, skinned

freshly ground black pepper

a little sea salt, if required

1 Heat the oil in a large, lidded pan or stockpot and add the onions, garlic and mushrooms. Sauté gently for about 5 minutes then stir in the coriander, cumin and ginger and cook for 2 minutes more.

2 Stir in the tomato purée and add the carrots and celery, stock, lentils and the chicken to the pan. Stir to ensure that the chicken is submerged in the liquid, then cover.

3 Simmer for 35 minutes, then uncover and simmer for a further 15 minutes or so more, as necessary, to let the sauce thicken and the chicken cook through – test a piece to see that the juices run clear.

4 Season with black pepper, taste to check the flavour and add a little sea salt if needed.

Cook's Notes

Allergy suitability: gluten/wheat/dairy/yeast free (depending on the stock)

Can be made in advance • Suitable for freezing

Health scores per serving: GL 7 • 🥕🥕🥕🥕🥕🥕 • BBB

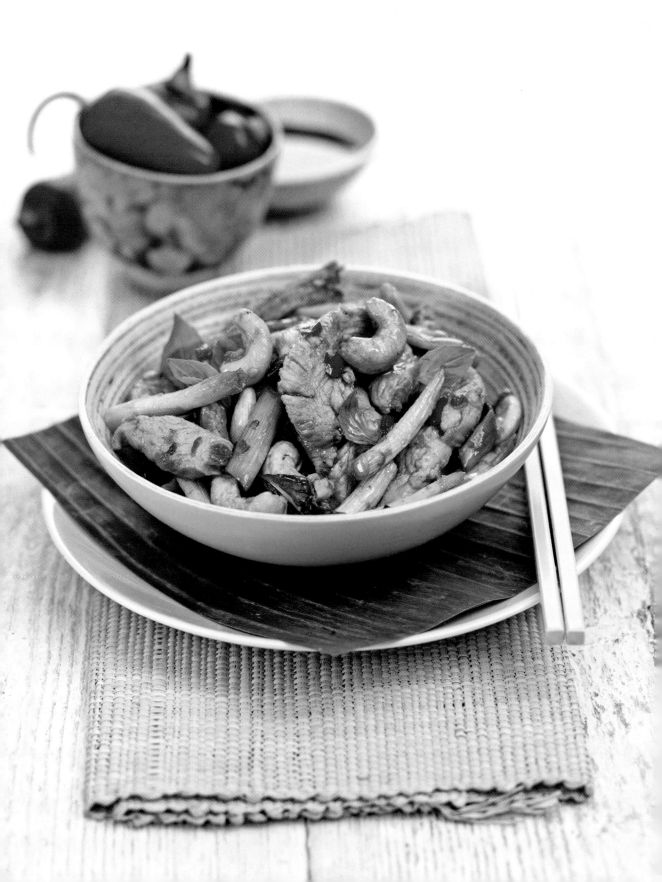

THAI CHICKEN AND CASHEW STIR-FRY

This is my husband Nick's dish. He grew up in Hong Kong and is a big fan of Asian-style food. Get all your ingredients fully prepped and ready to throw into the wok before you begin cooking, because this is fast and furious. It is too fast-cooking for steam-frying. Serve with brown basmati rice or soba (buckwheat) noodles, and perhaps some stir-fried greens – try the Stir-fried Choi Sum with Oyster Sauce on page 174. You can get holy basil leaves from Chinese supermarkets (don't substitute ordinary basil as the flavour is very different).

Serves 2

2 garlic cloves

2 small red chillies, deseeded

1½ tbsp mild flavoured oil such as rapeseed oil, or coconut oil

2 skinless chicken breasts, cut into thin strips

8 spring onions, trimmed and cut into 2.5cm (1in) strips on the diagonal

115g (4oz) roasted, unsalted cashew nuts

1 tsp xylitol (or white sugar)

2 tsp soy or tamari sauce

1½ tbsp fish sauce

3 tbsp chicken stock

15 holy basil leaves, shredded

1 tbsp Thai chilli paste

1 Crush the garlic and chillies to a paste.

2 Heat the wok until medium hot, then add the oil and swirl to coat the wok.

3 Add the garlic and chilli paste and chicken and cook for 2–3 minutes until the chicken is cooked.

4 Add the spring onions and cook for 30 seconds before adding the cashew nuts and cooking for another 30 seconds.

5 Add the xylitol or sugar, soy or tamari and fish sauce. Stir well, then add the stock.

6 Add the basil leaves and Thai chilli paste and stir before serving.

Cook's Notes

Allergy suitability: gluten/wheat/dairy free (depending on sauces, stock and chilli paste)

Health scores per serving: GL 5 • 🥕 • B B B

SLOW-COOKED PORK WITH WINTER VEGETABLES

This warming one-pot stew is packed with winter goodness from the root vegetables. Using celeriac will keep the GL lower than with potatoes, as celeriac contains much less starch. You could even add some kale while cooking, for extra methylation-supporting nutrients.

Serves 4

500g (1lb 2oz) pork shoulder, cut into chunks
cornflour to coat, seasoned with a little sea or
 rock salt
2 tbsp goose fat or a mild flavoured oil for
 frying, like olive or rapeseed
2 garlic cloves, crushed
2 leeks, thickly cut
2 carrots, thickly cut

6 small onions or shallots
575g (1lb 5oz) celeriac or potatoes, cut into
 chunks
200ml (7fl oz) strong chicken stock
200ml (7fl oz) white wine
large rosemary sprig
freshly ground black pepper

1 Preheat the oven to 120°C/250°F/Gas ½.

2 Roll the pork shoulder in the seasoned cornflour to coat.

3 Heat the fat or oil in a large, lidded, flameproof casserole or large ovenproof pan and brown the meat on all sides.

4 Add the garlic, leeks, carrots, whole onions and celeriac or potatoes to the pan, and stir.

5 Pour in the stock and wine, stir and dunk the rosemary into the mixture, then cover and bring to the boil.

6 Put the dish into the oven for 1 hour, then stir and cook for a further 1 hour, or until the pork is very tender and the vegetables are soft. Season with black pepper after cooking and remove the rosemary before serving.

Cook's Notes
Allergy suitability: gluten/wheat/dairy free (depending on the stock used) • Can be made in advance
• Suitable for freezing
Health scores per serving: GL 10 (using celeriac) • 🥕 • 𝔹𝔹𝔹

SHEPHERD'S PIE WITH SWEET POTATO TOPPING

My version of this winter classic replaces ordinary potatoes with sweet potatoes, which are less likely to upset blood sugar levels. Their vivid orange colour not only lends visual appeal to the dish but it is also an indication of the considerable antioxidant content of the sweet potato. This is a complete dish in its own right, with plenty of vegetables contained within the mince filling, but you could also serve it with some steamed savoy cabbage, cauliflower or broccoli.

Serves 4

500g (1lb 2oz) lamb mince
2 carrots, diced
2 garlic cloves, crushed
2 leeks, finely sliced
2 tbsp tomato purée
450ml (16fl oz) beef stock

splash of Worcestershire sauce
freshly ground black pepper
about 950g (2lb 2oz) sweet potatoes, cubed
a little olive or rapeseed oil, or a knob of butter
   for mashing

1 Preheat the oven to 180°C/350°F/Gas 4.

2 Brown the mince in a large, hot pan. Break up with a spoon, then add the carrots, garlic and leeks. Let them sauté a little for 5 minutes or so.

3 Stir in the tomato purée, stock and Worcestershire sauce. Bring to a simmer, then cover and cook for 20 minutes. Stir and cook for a further 20 minutes, uncovered.

4 Meanwhile, steam the sweet potatoes for 15 minutes or until tender. Mash with a little oil or butter, if you like.

5 Spoon the lamb mixture into an ovenproof dish and spread the mashed sweet potato evenly over the top. Ruffle the top with a fork, then bake for 20–25 minutes or until the top starts to colour and the mince is starting to bubble at the edges. You can pop it under the grill to get a golden brown colour if you wish.

Cook's Notes

Allergy suitability: wheat/dairy free (if you use oil in the mash) • Can be made in advance
Suitable for freezing
Health scores per serving: GL 9 • 🥕🥕🥕 • ⒷⒷⒷ

THAI LAMB RED CURRY

Don't be tempted to opt for reduced-fat coconut milk for this recipe: the fat is where all the goodness is found. Coconut milk is rich in medium-chain triglycerides or MCTs, which have been shown to have a host of health benefits, not least being used preferentially as energy rather than being stored as fat. Serve this full-flavoured curry with a mixture of brown basmati and wild rice. This recipe keeps well so it's good for a 'leftovers' dinner the following day.

Serves 6

1 tbsp coconut oil or virgin rapeseed oil

3 tbsp Thai red curry paste

900g (2lb) diced lamb leg

100g (3½oz) unsalted cashew nuts, blitzed in a food processor to finely chop

2 tbsp tomato purée

2 x 400ml cans full-fat coconut milk

4 Thai lime leaves, roughly crumbled (optional) (see Cook's Notes)

300g (10½oz) mangetout or fine green beans

2 tbsp Thai fish sauce

lime wedges, to serve

1 Heat the oil in a wok over a high heat. Add the curry paste and stir-fry for 1 minute then add the meat and stir-fry to coat it in the paste.

2 Tip the cashew nuts into the wok with the tomato purée, coconut milk and lime leaves, and bring to the boil. Reduce the heat slightly, cover and simmer, stirring occasionally, for about 50–60 minutes, or until the sauce has reduced and thickened.

3 Shortly before serving, boil or steam the mangetout or green beans until al dente, then stir into the curry along with the fish sauce. Serve with rice and lime wedges for squeezing.

Cook's Notes

You can buy Thai lime leaves freeze dried, but it is fine to omit them if you can't get hold of them.

Allergy suitability: gluten/wheat/dairy free (depending on curry paste and fish sauce)

Can be made in advance

Health scores per serving: GL 5 • B B B

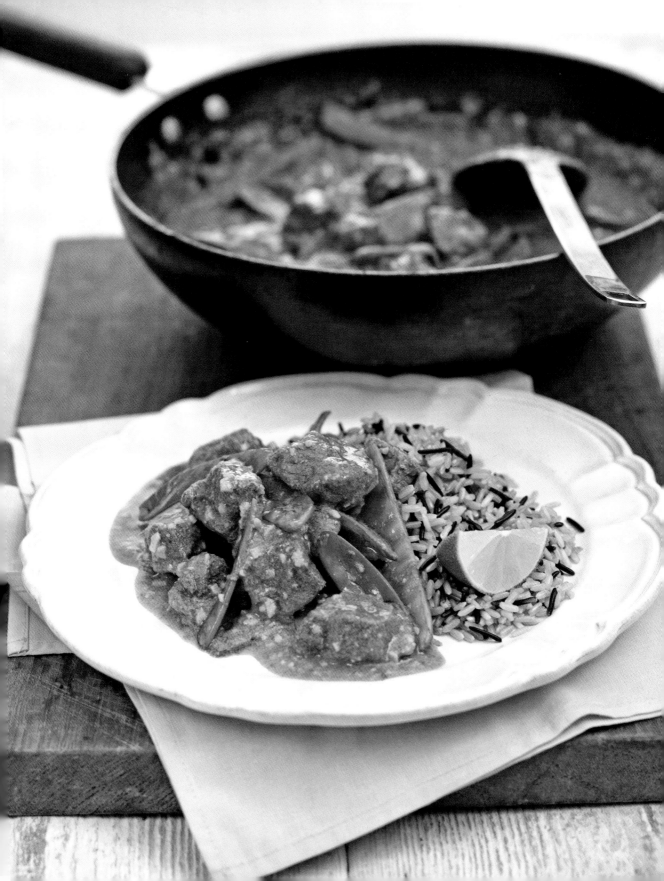

SIMPLE BEEF, ONION AND MUSHROOM STEW

Red wine lends flavonoid antioxidants as well as richness of flavour to this stew. Mushrooms are a good addition to stews or Bolognese-type dishes as they add bulk without starch, to help keep the GL of the dish low, and they are also rich in B vitamins. Serve with boiled or steamed baby new potatoes and the Braised Kale with Almonds on page 176.

Serves 4

450g (1lb) braising steak, cut into bite-sized cubes

2 tbsp cornflour, sprinkled over a plate and seasoned with sea or rock salt

mild or medium (not extra virgin) olive oil, virgin rapeseed oil or coconut oil

1 garlic clove, crushed

2 onions, sliced

350g (12oz) mushrooms, quartered (or use whole button mushrooms)

4 carrots, sliced

2 celery sticks, sliced

1 bay leaf

275ml (9½fl oz) beef stock

275ml (9½fl oz) red wine

freshly ground black pepper

sea or rock salt to taste

1 Preheat the oven to 150°C/300°F/Gas 2. Dust the beef on all sides with the seasoned cornflour. Heat a little oil in a frying pan, add the beef and brown on all sides, transferring to a casserole when done. Do this in stages, if necessary, to avoid overcrowding the meat in the pan.

2 Add more oil to the pan as necessary and fry the garlic, onions and mushrooms for about 5 minutes, then add to the casserole along with the carrots, celery, bay leaf and stock.

3 Pour the wine into the frying pan and bring to the boil, scraping off the sediment from the base of the pan as it bubbles. Pour it all over the meat and vegetables in the casserole.

4 Put the lid on the casserole and cook in the oven for about 2½ hours, stirring halfway. Season to taste and remove the bay leaf before serving.

Cook's Notes

Allergy suitability: gluten/wheat/dairy free (depending on stock used) • Can be made in advance
Health scores per serving: GL 4 • 🥕🥕🥕🥕🥕 • Ⓑ Ⓑ Ⓑ

PUMPKIN AND BACON ONE POT

This dish can be on the table in half an hour flat and is absolutely delicious, bursting with hearty flavours that are perfect for a winter supper. It is bowl food at its best. The cruciferous green veg and the carotene-rich pumpkin or squash also serve to offset the fact that bacon is not top of the list of recommended foods – but by serving it in a stew, a little goes a long way.

Serves 4

200g (7oz) streaky bacon, chopped

about 850g (1lb 14oz) pumpkin or squash, cubed

1 large red onion, sliced into thin wedges

300ml (10fl oz/½ pint) hot chicken stock

1 head spring greens, Brussel tops or kale, very finely sliced

freshly ground black pepper

1 Heat a large frying pan, add the bacon and fry until brown and starting to crisp.

2 Add the pumpkin and onion and let them sauté to allow the pumpkin to pick up some colour.

3 Pour in the stock, bring to the boil, then cover and simmer for about 15 minutes so that the pumpkin cooks and becomes tender.

4 Add the greens, cover and simmer for a further 5 minutes or so until they become tender.

5 Sprinkle with black pepper before serving.

Cook's Notes

Allergy suitability: gluten/wheat/dairy/yeast free (depending on stock used)

Can be made in advance

Health scores per serving: GL 8 • *↑↑↑* • B B B

VENISON AND CHOCOLATE STEW

Chocolate complements gamey venison and by using cacao (raw chocolate) or dark, high-cocoa, solid chocolate you can substantially increase the ORAC value. Serve with spring greens or cabbage.

Serves 4

75g (3oz) streaky bacon, diced, or smoked bacon lardons (optional)

600g (1lb 5oz) diced venison stewing steak (haunch, neck or shoulder)

2 tbsp seasoned plain flour

mild or medium (not extra virgin) olive oil, or virgin rapeseed oil, for frying

150g (5½oz) shallots, coarsely chopped

2 garlic cloves, sliced

1 celery stick, finely chopped

2 carrots, finely chopped

2 thyme sprigs

2 rosemary sprigs

1 glass red wine, about 250ml (9fl oz)

2 tbsp tomato purée

300ml (10fl oz/½ pint) hot chicken, beef or vegetable stock

30g/1¼oz dried wild mushrooms, soaked for 20 minutes or according to pack instructions

2 bay leaves

sprinkle of sea or rock salt

freshly ground black pepper

20g/¾oz cacao or decent dark chocolate

handful fresh flat-leaf parsley, chopped

1 Preheat the oven to 160°C/325°F/Gas 3. Fry the bacon, if using, in a frying pan, then remove from the pan. Clean the pan if it was sticking.

2 Put the venison and seasoned flour into a clean plastic food bag or freezer bag and shake to coat. Remove any excess flour.

3 Add some oil for frying to the pan, add the meat and brown (in batches if necessary).

4 Remove the meat and add the shallots and garlic to the pan. Fry for 2 minutes then add the celery, carrots and herbs. Cook for a further 5 minutes.

5 Return the meat and bacon to the pan and add the wine to deglaze.

6 Add the tomato purée, stock, mushrooms, bay leaves and seasoning. Bring to the boil then cook in the preheated oven for 1½–2 hours until the meat is meltingly tender. Remove the herb sprigs and bay leaves and stir in the cacao or chocolate, plus parsley. Check the seasoning before serving.

Cook's Notes

Allergy suitability: gluten/wheat/dairy free (depending on stock)

Can be made in advance • Suitable for freezing

Health scores per serving: GL 2 • 🥕🥕🥕🥕 • B B B

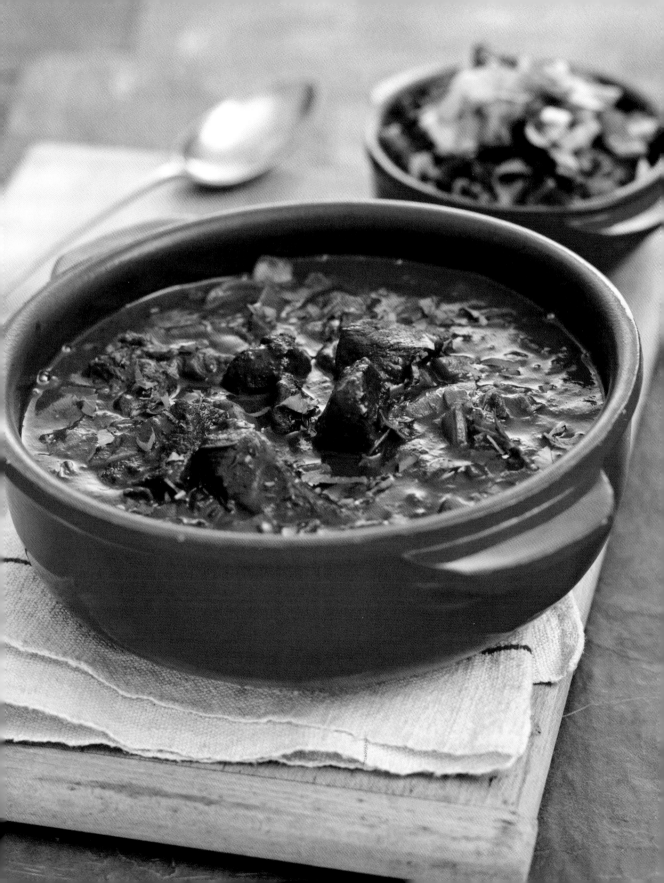

CUMIN-SPICED MEATBALLS

By simply rolling these little beef patties in cumin, you not only add considerable flavour, thus reducing the amount of salt they will require, but this will also add hugely to the ORAC score. Here I have combined them with the Bean and Mushroom Bolognese recipe on page 154, a pairing that is particularly good served with wholemeal spaghetti and perhaps a green salad. However, they could equally be served without the bolognese in a wholemeal pitta with hummus and coleslaw.

Serves 4

500g (1lb 2oz) beef mince
good sprinkle of sea or rock salt
plenty of freshly ground black pepper
about 3 tbsp ground cumin

2 tbsp mild or medium olive oil, or virgin
   rapeseed oil
1 quantity Bean and Mushroom Bolognese (see
   page 154)

1 Press the mince out flat on a chopping board to break it up. Season generously with salt and pepper. Bring the mince together and repeat the process to ensure that the meatballs will be evenly and adequately seasoned.

2 Roll the mince into 24 balls, each roughly the size of a walnut.

3 Sprinkle the cumin onto a plate and roll each meatball over the cumin to lightly coat.

4 Heat the oil in a large frying pan until hot, then add the meatballs and cook for about 5 minutes, moving them about steadily, until browned evenly on all sides.

5 Add the Bean and Mushroom Bolognese and let the meatballs simmer in the sauce for a further 8 minutes or until cooked through and the middle is not too pink.

Cook's Notes

Allergy suitability: gluten/wheat/dairy/yeast free • Can be made in advance
Suitable for freezing (freeze after step 2, before coating in cumin and cooking)
Health scores per serving: GL 1 • 🥕🥕🥕🥕🥕 • Ⓑ

QUINOA JAMBALAYA

In this version of a Caribbean jambalaya I have replaced rice with quinoa, to make this considerably lower GL and higher in valuable minerals such as calcium and zinc. You can vary this recipe endlessly, much like a paella or risotto, but whichever meat or fish you choose to use, try to ensure that you have a good range of different coloured vegetables, to maximise the antioxidant content.

Serves 4

1 tbsp mild or medium (not extra virgin) olive oil, virgin rapeseed oil or coconut oil
2 onions, sliced
2 garlic cloves, crushed
2 red peppers, deseeded and thinly sliced
2 celery sticks, thinly sliced
4 tsp Cajun spice/jerk seasoning blend

150g (5½oz) good-quality smoked sausage, such as Hungarian Mangalica paprika, sliced (see Cook's Notes)
750ml (1¼ pints) pork or chicken stock
175g (6oz) quinoa, rinsed and drained
good-sized bunch flat-leaf parsley, finely chopped
squeeze of lemon or lime juice to serve (optional)

1 Heat the oil in a large, lidded pan, add the onions, garlic, peppers, celery and Cajun spices and sauté for 15 minutes.

2 Stir in the sausage and fry for 2 minutes to colour slightly, then pour in the stock. Bring to the boil before adding the quinoa.

3 Reduce to a simmer over very low heat, cover and cook for about 20 minutes, uncovering after the first 10 minutes to allow the liquid to reduce.

4 Stir the parsley through the quinoa and taste to check the flavours. Squeeze some lemon or lime juice over the top, if you like.

Cook's Notes

When choosing the smoked sausage, avoid the cheaper, additive-ridden brands.
Allergy suitability: gluten/wheat/dairy free (depending on the contents of the stock and sausage)
Can be made in advance
Health scores per serving: GL 4 • B B B

FISH

SOME PEOPLE TEND TO SHY away from cooking fish, under the misapprehension that it is difficult. In fact I think fish is the very definition of fast food. Time-poor people getting back from work could cook a salmon fillet, for example, and throw some bagged salad onto a plate faster than you could cook pasta or pizza. I hope that this section therefore provides suitable inspiration and easy recipes to encourage reluctant fish eaters to try to include this wonder food more often in their menus. I have included a lot of oily fish in these recipes in a bid to help you meet your weekly omega-3 requirements as set out in Part One. These are clearly marked in the Cook's Notes to make it easy for you to keep track, denoted with a Ω. Your goal, for optimal health, is to achieve $\Omega\,\Omega\,\Omega$ a day. One serving of oily fish gives you three, while a serving of white fish gives you two. Lastly, I have also included some of the increasingly popular white fish, like tilapia, which I think is an excellent alternative to cod, being easy to cook, firm fleshed and mild in flavour. Children and people who are not keen on very 'fishy' fish seem to find it far more palatable.

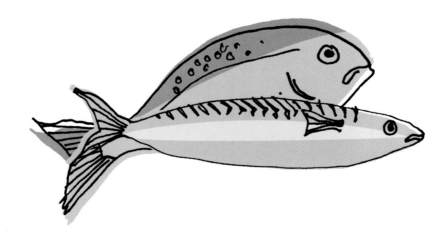

BAKED TROUT WITH LEMON AND ALMONDS

This version of the French classic is baked rather than grilled, to preserve more of the valuable omega-3 fats and also to retain more moisture in the fish. It is meltingly soft and delicious served with boiled new potatoes and a green leaf salad.

Serves 2

2 trout fillets (about 225g/8oz each), gutted and rinsed

1 unwaxed or organic lemon, halved, ends removed, then cut into thin slices

60g (2oz) butter

35g/1¼oz flaked almonds

1 tbsp fresh lemon juice

2 tbsp finely chopped flat-leaf parsley

pinch sea or rock salt

freshly ground black pepper

1 Preheat the oven to 200°C/400°F/Gas 6. You will need a shallow ovenproof dish large enough to accommodate the fish fillets in one layer.

2 Carefully cut diagonal slashes about 5mm (¼in) deep into both sides of each fish. Put the fish side by side in the dish and tuck the halved lemon slices into the slashes.

3 Gently melt half the butter in a small pan, taking care not to let it boil. Spoon half of it over the fish fillets, then put the dish in the preheated oven to cook, uncovered, for 20 minutes, or until the fish flakes easily when pressed with a fork.

4 Toast the almonds in a dry frying pan until just turning golden, then take off the heat, immediately throw in the remaining butter and let it sizzle to melt. Quickly tip in the lemon juice and season with salt, pepper and parsley. Taste to adjust the seasoning as necessary.

5 Put the fish onto plates and spoon on some of the juice from the dish and the almond butter sauce over the top of each. Serve immediately.

Cook's Notes

Allergy suitability: gluten/wheat/yeast free

Health scores per serving: GL 0 • $\Omega\,\Omega$ • $\boxed{B}\,\boxed{B}$

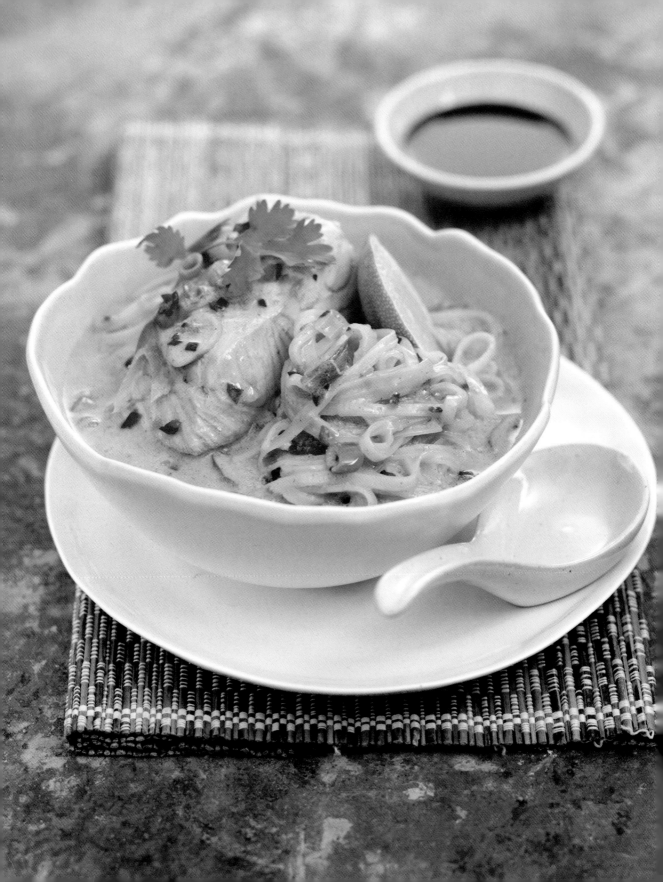

THAI SALMON NOODLE BOWL

The flavours of spring onions, chilli, curry spices and lime add considerable antioxidants as well as flavour to this take on Asian bowl food. Plus, of course, the salmon provides omega-3 essential fats.

Serves 2

1 tbsp virgin rapeseed oil

2 spring onions, finely sliced on the diagonal

1 red chilli, deseeded and very finely chopped

2 tbsp Thai red curry paste

165ml can full-fat coconut milk

500ml (18fl oz) chicken stock

2 skinless salmon fillets, about 125g (4½oz) each

115g (4oz) noodles (ideally a lower GL variety, like soba or brown rice noodles)

1 tbsp fish sauce

juice of 1 lime

a few coriander leaves, to garnish

1 Heat the oil in a frying pan or wok. Add the spring onions and chilli and stir-fry for 1 minute. Stir in the curry paste and cook for 2 minutes or until fragrant.

2 Add the coconut milk and stock, and simmer for 5 minutes. Reduce the heat and add the fish. Poach for 4–5 minutes or until just cooked – the flesh should flake easily when pressed.

3 Cook the noodles according to the pack instructions. Drain and divide between two soup bowls, twisting about a fork so that they lie in a neat circle.

4 Put a salmon fillet on top of the noodles in each bowl.

5 Add the fish sauce and lime juice to the soup and pour over the noodles. Top with the coriander.

Cook's Notes

Allergy suitability: gluten/wheat/dairy/yeast free (depending on the Thai paste and stock)

Health scores per serving: GL 8 • $\Omega\,\Omega\,\Omega$ • B

STEAMED TROUT WITH GINGER

This is quick to prepare and to cook, full of Asian flavours but light on calories. The addition of chilli, ginger, garlic and lime makes a simple steamed fish dish much more interesting, as well as contributing antioxidants and a myriad of other health benefits. Try serving this dish with brown basmati rice or soba (buckwheat) noodles tossed with toasted sesame seeds.

Serves 2

2 trout fillets, each weighing about 140g (5oz)

115g (4oz) baby pak choi, each quartered lengthways

3 spring onions, finely sliced on the diagonal

1 small garlic clove, crushed

1 tsp very finely chopped fresh root ginger

1 tsp red chilli, deseeded and very finely chopped

grated zest and juice of 1 lime

2 tbsp tamari or soy sauce

1 tbsp toasted sesame oil

1 Cut a large rectangle of baking parchment. Put into a steamer pan, then put the fish fillets next to each other in the middle of the paper.

2 Put the pak choi around the edge of the fish and scatter the spring onions over the top.

3 Mix the garlic, ginger, chilli, lime juice and zest, tamari or soy and sesame oil together in a small bowl or cup and pour over the fish and vegetables.

4 Bring the edges of the paper together in the middle and fold over to loosely seal. Steam the parcel for 15 minutes.

5 Open the parcel carefully, check that the fish is cooked by pressing to see if it flakes easily, then spoon onto plates.

Cook's Notes

Allergy suitability: gluten/wheat/dairy free (depending on soy sauce)

Can be made in advance (chill the parcels in the fridge before cooking)

Health scores per serving: GL 0 • $\Omega\,\Omega\,\Omega$ • B B B

PATRICK'S SUPER-HEALTHY KEDGEREE

Not a kedgeree for purists, but no less delicious for it. We have gone for broke here by using plenty of high-ORAC-scoring spices and Tenderstem broccoli. We have also replaced white rice with brown and reduced the proportion of rice to other goodies in a bid to keep the GL of the dish as low as possible.

Serves 4

175g (6oz) brown basmati rice

1 large undyed smoked haddock fillet, about 275g (10oz)

2 free-range or organic eggs

200g (7oz) Tenderstem broccoli

115g (4oz) frozen petit pois

2 tbsp mild, medium (not extra virgin) olive oil, virgin rapeseed oil or coconut oil

1 garlic clove, crushed

1 large or 2 small onions, finely chopped

1 tbsp mild curry powder

1 tsp ground turmeric

4 tbsp finely chopped flat-leaf parsley

freshly ground black pepper

a little sea salt, if required

lemons wedges, to serve

1 Cook the rice according to the pack instructions, then drain and keep warm until ready to use.

2 Meanwhile, fill a large frying pan with water and bring to a gentle boil. Put the haddock in the pan, making sure it is covered by the liquid, and gently poach for 4–6 minutes or until the flesh flakes easily when pressed. Carefully remove the fish from the pan and leave to cool. Then remove the skin and flake into pieces, picking out any bones.

3 Hard-boil the eggs in a pan of boiling water for 6 minutes then cool rapidly under the tap for 1 minute. Set aside to fully cool before peeling and slicing into quarters.

4 Steam the broccoli and petit pois for about 3 minutes, then slice the broccoli.

5 Add the oil to a large pan, add the garlic and onion and sauté for 1 minute or so before adding the spices. Cook gently for a further few minutes, until the onions are soft and fragrant.

6 Stir the cooked rice into the onion and spice mixture until evenly coated. Gently fold in the flaked haddock, broccoli, peas and hard-boiled eggs.

7 Season with plenty of pepper – you may not need any salt. Add the parsley and stir carefully. Taste to check the seasoning and serve with a lemon wedge on each plate.

Cook's Notes

Allergy suitability: gluten/wheat/dairy/yeast free • Can be made in advance

Health scores per serving: GL 8 • 🥕🥕🥕🥕 • ΩΩ • BBB

STEAMED SALMON WITH SOY AND GARLIC SPRING GREENS

Steaming is perhaps the healthiest method of all for cooking oily fish, as it is so gentle on the delicate essential fats. It can be a little dull, however, so here I have used stir-fried soy and garlic greens to enliven the flavour. Have everything ready before you start, as this recipe relies upon working quickly to serve everything as soon as possible after cooking.

Serves 2

2 salmon fillets, about 110g (3¾oz) each

2 tsp tamari or soy sauce

2 tbsp groundnut oil, or virgin rapeseed oil

6 spring onions, very finely sliced lengthways

For the spring greens

2 tbsp virgin rapeseed oil or coconut oil

2 garlic cloves, lightly crushed using the back of the knife and kept whole

2 small heads of spring greens, thinly sliced horizontally (see Cook's Notes)

2 tsp tamari or soy sauce, or to taste

1 Steam the salmon for 10–14 minutes depending on size, until the flesh flakes readily when pressed.

2 Meanwhile, cook the spring greens. Add the oil to a hot wok or frying pan, add the garlic, stir-fry for about 15 seconds then add the greens and stir-fry for a further 2 minutes to let them soften slightly. Add the tamari or soy sauce, stir and taste, then set to one side as you quickly serve the fish.

3 Put the salmon fillets onto two plates and drizzle with a teaspoon of tamari or soy sauce.

4 Heat the oil in a frying pan until very hot, then throw in the spring onions and cook for about 1 minute to just wilt. Spoon the spring onions over each piece of salmon.

Cook's Notes

When cutting the spring greens, slice almost as far as the central stalk, as this is the sweetest part.

Allergy suitability: gluten/wheat/dairy/yeast free (depending on tamari or soy used)

Health scores per serving: GL 1 • $\Omega\Omega\Omega$ • B̄B̄

SMOKED PAPRIKA-SPICED TILAPIA WITH TENDERSTEM BROCCOLI

Tilapia is a great choice for anyone looking for a sustainable replacement for cod, whiting or haddock, and British fish farmers are starting to establish tilapia farms, so in the future it may not have to come from Africa. It has a delicate flavour and texture which works well with the strong, smoky paprika in this recipe. Serve with baby new potatoes.

Serves 2

1 tbsp mild or medium (not extra virgin) olive oil, or virgin rapeseed oil

1 tsp smoked paprika

2 tilapia fillets

200g (7oz) Tenderstem broccoli

good pinch sea or rock salt

freshly ground black pepper

2 lemon wedges

1 Stir the oil, paprika and salt together on a plate, then coat both sides of the fish fillets in the mixture.

2 Heat a large frying pan to a high heat and add the fish (pans that are not non-stick may need a little extra oil). Cook for about 3 minutes on each side or until the flesh flakes easily when pressed. Meanwhile, steam the broccoli for about 3 minutes.

3 Sprinkle the cooked fish with black pepper and serve with the broccoli and a wedge of lemon.

Cook's Notes

Allergy suitability: gluten/wheat/dairy/yeast free

Health scores per serving: GL 3 • 🥕🥕 • ΩΩ • B̄ B̄

GARLIC CHILLI PRAWNS WITH PAK CHOI

I am not usually a fan of prawns, but this dish has me converted. The strong citrus, chilli and garlic flavours make this an aromatic treat. The prawns take 3 minutes to cook, so make sure you have the pak choi ready to go as soon as they come off the heat. Serve with brown basmati rice.

Serves 2

3 garlic cloves, crushed

juice of 2 limes

1 green chilli, deseeded

1 spoonful chilli-infused oil (from Chinese supermarkets), or a pinch of dried chilli flakes

good pinch of rock or sea salt

3 tbsp virgin rapeseed oil

300g (11oz) large fresh, raw prawns, fully prepared

1 Put the garlic in a blender with the lime juice, chilli, chilli oil or chilli flakes, salt and oil. Whiz to a purée.

2 Marinate the prepared prawns in this mixture for 20 minutes at room temperature.

3 Cook for 1½ minutes per side on a medium hot griddle or frying pan.

4 To cook the pak choi, add the oil to a hot wok or frying pan and stir-fry or steam-fry (by adding a dash of water and then covering) the pak choi stems for 1 minute, then add the leaves and cook for about 3 minutes, or until just cooked.

5 Remove from the heat and stir the oyster sauce through the pak choi.

6 Serve immediately with the prawns.

Cook's Notes

Allergy suitability: wheat/dairy/yeast free (depending on oyster sauce)

Health scores per serving: GL 1 • ⚕ • B B

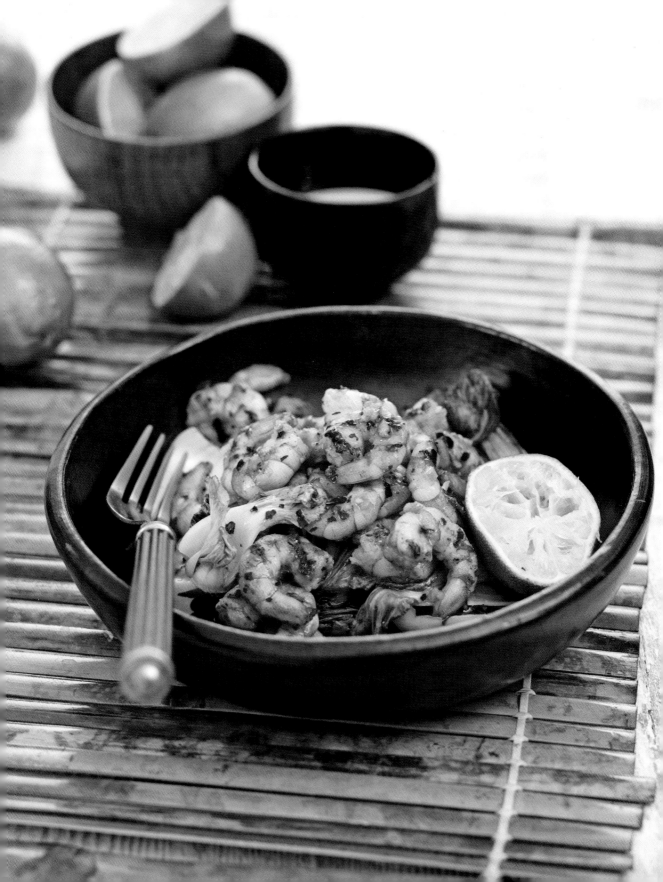

PAN-FRIED POLLOCK AND SWEET POTATO CHIPS

A healthier take on the great British takeaway. Sweet potato appears to help your body regulate blood sugar levels, making it a much better choice for your chips than ordinary white potatoes. Serve with a green leaf salad or some wilted spinach.

Serves 2

2 pollock fillets, about 150g (5½oz) each, preferably with skin on

1 tbsp mild or medium olive oil or virgin rapeseed oil

a little sea or rock salt

freshly ground black pepper

2 lemon wedges, to serve

For the chips

1 medium-large sweet potato, cut into chips

1 tbsp mild or medium olive oil or virgin rapeseed oil

a little sea or rock salt

1 Heat oven to 180°C/350°F/Gas 4.

2 To cook the chips, toss the sweet potato chips with the oil and a little salt.

3 Spread out in a shallow roasting tin and roast for 30–40 minutes or until crisp.

4 Lightly sprinkle the fish fillets with a little salt. Heat the oil in a medium hot frying pan, then put the fish in the pan, skin side down at first. Cook the fish for 2 minutes or so, until the fillets are opaque almost all the way through. Turn the fish over and carry on cooking until the fish has coloured all of the way through (this will only take another minute or so).

5 Put the fish on plates with the sweet potato chips and season with black pepper. Serve with a lemon wedge.

Cook's Notes

Allergy suitability: gluten/wheat/dairy/yeast free

Health scores per serving: GL 7 • $\Omega\Omega$ • $\boxed{B}\boxed{B}$

FISH MEDLEY IN A WHITE SAUCE

This fish dish is very versatile. Dollop some crushed new potatoes on top for an instant fish pie or serve with rice and peas. The milk and butter substitutions also make this easy to adapt for people avoiding dairy products.

Serves 4

600ml (20fl oz/1 pint) milk, or non-dairy milk

650g (1lb 7oz) fish pie mix (see Cook's Notes)

3 leeks, sliced

25g (1oz) butter or non-dairy spread suitable for cooking, plus a little extra for frying

25g (1oz) plain flour

2 tbsp finely chopped flat-leaf parsley

a little sea or rock salt, if you like

white pepper

1 Put the milk in a large frying pan and heat so that bubbles just begin to appear. Add the fish and gently poach for about 8 minutes, or until it flakes easily when pressed.

2 Remove from the pan and put on a plate, reserving the milk to make the sauce.

3 Fry the leeks in a little extra butter or oil, sautéing for about 5 minutes or until soft.

4 Make the white sauce by melting the 25g/1oz butter in a pan, then stir in the flour and cook for 1–2 minutes. Take off the heat and gradually stir in the milk so that it becomes a smooth mixture.

5 Return to the heat and, stirring constantly, bring to the boil, then reduce the heat and simmer for 8–10 minutes, or until it has thickened, stirring from time to time.

6 Fold the fish, leeks, pepper and parsley into the white sauce. Season to taste – the fish will add flavour and salt to the sauce – and serve with your chosen accompaniment.

Cook's Notes

You can buy fish pie mix at your supermarket fish counter. This is prepared bite-sized pieces of fish, such as salmon, haddock and pollock. If unavailable, buy a mixture of white and oily fish, for example some salmon, haddock and pollock.

Allergy suitability: dairy/yeast free (if using non-dairy alternatives)

Can be made in advance • Suitable for freezing

Health scores per serving: GL 7 • $\Omega\,\Omega\,\Omega$ • $\boxed{B}\,\boxed{B}$

MONKFISH WRAPPED IN PARMA HAM

The Parma ham adds a little fat, which helps to stop the monkfish from drying out during cooking. This is delicious served with the Herby Puy Lentils on page 169. Alternatively try it with and the Peperonata on page 173 for a Mediterranean-inspired meal.

Serves 2

2 monkfish fillets, about 175g (6oz) each
freshly ground black pepper
4 slices Parma ham

1 tbsp mild or medium virgin olive oil, rapeseed
   or avocado oil
lemon wedges, to serve

1 Preheat the oven to 200°C/400°F/Gas 6.

2 Sprinkle black pepper over the monkfish to season, then wrap each fillet in a slice or two of Parma ham, to cover.

3 Place on a baking tray, drizzle with the oil and bake for 20 minutes. Squeeze lemon juice over before serving.

Cook's Notes

Allergy suitability: gluten/wheat/dairy/yeast free
Can be made in advance (pop the fillets in the fridge before cooking)
Health scores per serving: GL 0 • $\Omega\,\Omega$ • $\boxed{\text{B}}$

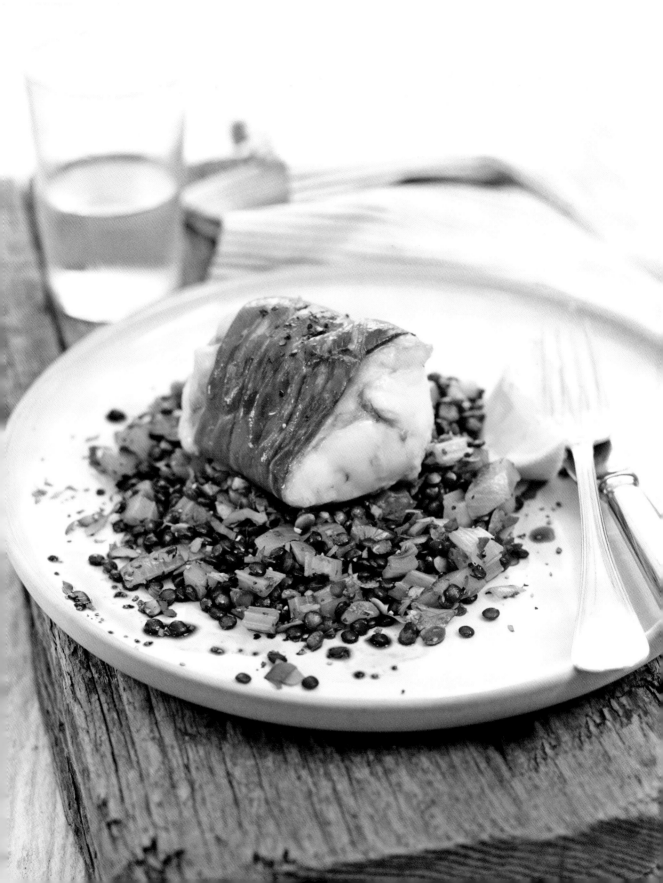

OMELETTE WITH SMOKED HADDOCK, PARMESAN AND CHIVES

The inspiration behind this dish was the classic Omelette Arnold Bennett, and I have tried to keep the same flavours but make it suitable for people trying to limit dairy products by removing the cream. Omit the Parmesan too, if you prefer. Serve with boiled baby new potatoes and a green salad.

Serves 2

1 large undyed smoked haddock fillet, about 275g/10oz
6 organic or free-range eggs
pinch of sea or rock salt

20g/¾oz butter or non-dairy spread suitable for cooking, or coconut oil
a little freshly grated Parmesan, optional
freshly ground black pepper
1 tbsp finely chopped fresh chives, to garnish

1 Fill a large frying pan with water and bring to a gentle boil. Put the haddock in the pan, making sure it is covered by the liquid, and poach for 3–4 minutes, until the fish flakes easily when pressed.

2 Carefully lift the fish onto a plate, drain off any excess liquid and set aside to cool, then flake into pieces, removing any skin or bones as you do so.

3 Preheat the grill to high. Break the eggs into a bowl and whisk with a pinch of salt.

4 Heat a frying pan (one that can be used under the grill) over a medium heat, add the butter or oil and move it about the pan to coat the base and sides, then pour in the eggs. As the omelette starts to set, repeatedly run the back of a fork across the base of the pan to lift up some of the mixture and let the uncooked egg spill underneath and cook.

5 Take the omelette off the heat when it has set on the bottom but the top is still very runny. Scatter the flaked fish over the omelette, then sprinkle with Parmesan, if using, and pop the pan under the grill for 2 minutes, watching constantly, until it starts to pick up a little colour and the top sets. Slide the omelette onto a plate, sprinkle with pepper and chives then cut in half and serve.

Cook's Notes

Allergy suitability: gluten/wheat/dairy/yeast free (if using dairy-free options)
Health scores per serving: GL 0 • $\Omega\,\Omega$ • $\boxed{B}\,\boxed{B}$

VEGETARIAN

WHETHER YOU ARE A COMMITTED VEGETARIAN or vegan or you simply want to reduce your meat intake and include more plant-based meals in your diet, this section should have plenty to suit you. The recipes follow the principles established in Part One, including plenty of low-GL starches like lentils, sweet potatoes and wild rice, combined with a rich variety of vegetables, herbs and spices to provide flavour, fibre and antioxidants. The dishes also provide protein, to ensure that you are consuming a suitably wide and balanced intake of the different essential amino acids. In response to feedback on previous cookbooks I have made a conscious effort to restrict the use of cheese, so you will find goat's cheese (which is easier to digest than cow's milk cheeses) in the Baked Sweet Potato dish on page 162, and the option of sprinkling Parmesan over the Celeriac and Artichoke Frittata on page 159, but other than that this is a cheese-free section, which I hope makes this more user-friendly for those avoiding dairy products.

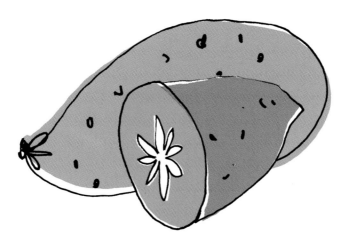

VEGETABLE STEAM-FRY

Serve this vegetable-rich steam-fry with quinoa if you want to boost the protein content and keep the GL score low, or with rice or noodles, watching the serving size to fit with your GL needs. Vary the vegetables according to taste but try to include a range of different colours so that you benefit from the full spectrum of antioxidants. You could also add ginger for an extra antioxidant boost.

Serves 2

1 tbsp virgin rapeseed oil or coconut oil
2 garlic cloves, finely sliced
½ red chilli, or to taste, deseeded and finely chopped
1 bunch spring onions, finely sliced
75g (3oz) unsalted cashew nuts
1 tbsp tamari or soy sauce

1 tbsp mirin
1 tbsp rice vinegar
1 small-medium carrot, julienned
2 heads of pak choi, sliced
200g (7oz) beansprouts
100ml (3½fl oz) vegetable stock, if needed

1 Heat the oil in a hot wok, swirl it about to coat the base and sides, then throw in the garlic, chilli, spring onions and cashew nuts and stir-fry for about 10 seconds before adding the tamari or soy sauce, mirin and rice vinegar.

2 Add the carrot, pak choi and beansprouts, and cover with a lid (or 2 sheets of kitchen paper doused in water if your wok does not have a lid) to let the vegetables steam-fry for 2 minutes or until al dente, adding the stock to keep it moist if necessary.

3 Remove the kitchen paper, stir and taste to check the seasoning.

Cook's Notes
Allergy suitability: gluten/wheat/dairy free (depending on soy or tamari and stock used) • V
Health scores per serving: GL 1 • 🥕 • Ⓑ Ⓑ Ⓑ

LENTIL DAHL

There are countless recipes for this Indian staple, which is traditionally served as a milder accompaniment to curries, but if you add plenty of spices, garlic and ginger it is very good served on its own with rice and perhaps some finely diced red onion, tomato and cucumber. The spices and garlic and ginger give this dish a very high ORAC score.

Serves 4

1 tbsp virgin rapeseed oil or coconut oil
1 tsp ground turmeric
1 tsp ground cumin
2 tsp garam masala
1 garlic clove, crushed
1 red onion, diced
2 tsp finely chopped fresh root ginger
1 medium carrot, diced or thinly sliced

165g (5¾oz) red lentils, rinsed and drained
750ml (1¼ pints) vegetable stock
1 medium sweet potato, cubed into small pieces
  (see Cook's Notes)
2 handfuls baby spinach, shredded
juice of ½ lemon
freshly ground black pepper
a little sea or rock salt

1 Heat the oil in a large frying pan, add the spices, garlic, onion and ginger and fry for 1 minute. Add the carrot and lentils, stir and pour in the stock.

2 Bring to the boil, then fast boil for 10 minutes before reducing the heat to a simmer. Add the sweet potato, stir, and cook for a further 15 minutes or until the lentils and sweet potato are soft.

3 Stir in the spinach and let it wilt, then add the lemon juice and season to taste before serving.

Cook's Notes

Peel the sweet potato if you prefer the look and texture of it, otherwise leave it unpeeled.

Allergy suitability: gluten/wheat/dairy/yeast free (depending on stock) • V

Can be made in advance • Suitable for freezing

Health scores per serving: GL 6 • 🥕🥕🥕🥕 • B B B

BEAN AND MUSHROOM BOLOGNESE

This thick, hearty bean stew works well with pasta and a rocket, watercress and spinach salad. The beans and mushrooms make it high in B vitamins. If you cannot get hold of pinto beans, borlotti beans are also delicious.

Serves 4

2 tbsp mild or medium olive oil, virgin rapeseed oil or coconut oil

1 large red onion, diced

2 garlic cloves, crushed

350g (12oz) mushrooms, thinly sliced

350g (12oz) tomato passata

400g can pinto beans, rinsed and drained

2 tsp vegetable bouillon powder

2 tsp dried oregano

freshly ground black pepper

1 Heat the oil in a large pan, add the onion and garlic and sauté for 10 minutes to soften. Add the mushrooms and cook for a further 5 minutes.

2 Pour in the passata, beans, bouillon and oregano, and bring up to a simmer. Cover and cook for 20 minutes or until the tomato has reduced slightly and the vegetables are soft.

3 Season to taste.

Cook's Notes

Allergy suitability: gluten/wheat/dairy/yeast free (depending on bouillon used)

V • Can be made in advance • Suitable for freezing

Health scores per serving: GL 7 • 🥕🥕🥕🥕🥕 • Ⓑ Ⓑ Ⓑ

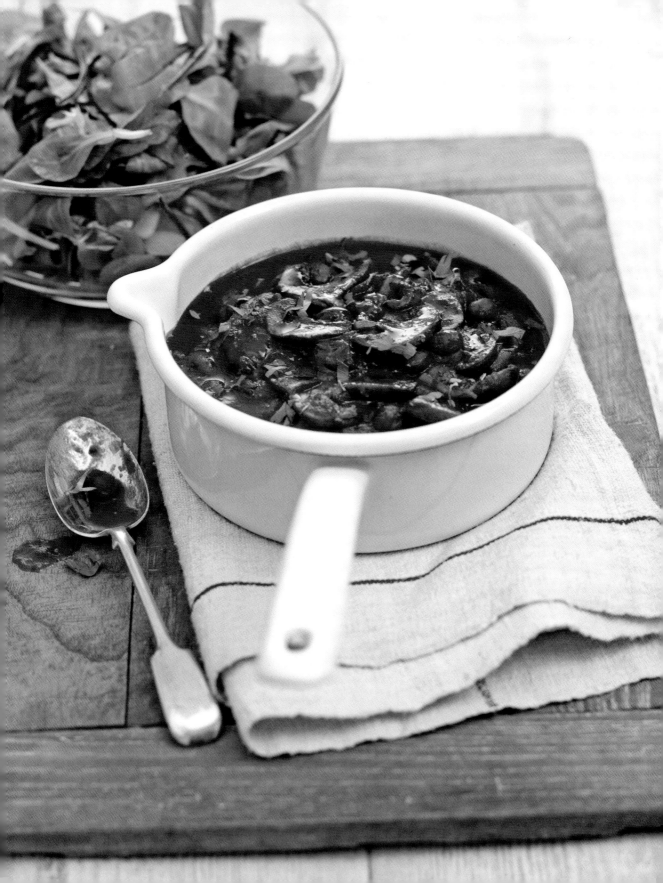

SWEET POTATO AND CHICKPEA STEW

My thanks to my good friend Nicky for providing the inspiration for this warming recipe. You can also use pumpkin or squash instead of sweet potato if you prefer. Serve with a mixture of brown basmati and wild rice, and/or a green salad, if you like.

Serves 4

1 tbsp mild or medium olive oil, virgin rapeseed oil or coconut oil

1 red onion, finely sliced

1 garlic clove, crushed

1 tsp finely chopped fresh root ginger

½ red chilli, deseeded and finely chopped

1 tsp turmeric

½ tsp smoked paprika

1 large sweet potato, unpeeled, diced (see Cook's Notes)

1 red pepper, thinly diced

400g can chickpeas, rinsed and drained

400g can chopped tomatoes

150ml (5fl oz/¼ pint) vegetable stock

freshly ground black pepper

a little sea or rock salt, to taste, if necessary

squeeze of lemon juice, to serve

1 Heat the oil in a large pan, add the onion and sauté for 10 minutes.

2 Add the garlic, ginger, chilli, turmeric and smoked paprika, and stir for 1 minute.

3 Add the sweet potato and pepper and cook for a further 5 minutes to let the vegetables start to colour.

4 Pour in the chickpeas, tomatoes and stock. Bring to the boil, then reduce the heat, cover and simmer gently for 20 minutes or until the sweet potato is tender.

5 Season to taste and squeeze some fresh lemon juice over the top before serving, to add extra pep and also to help lower the GL score.

Cook's Notes

Do peel the sweet potato if you are serving this to guests and want it to look a bit prettier.

Allergy suitability: gluten/wheat/dairy/yeast free (depending on the stock) • V

Can be made in advance • Suitable for freezing

Health scores per serving: GL 8 • 🥕 • 𝔹𝔹𝔹

QUINOA PILAF WITH RED PEPPER AND PUMPKIN SEEDS

This pilaf has a much lower GL than you could expect from the traditional rice-based version, thanks to the high-protein, low-starch quinoa. Quinoa is also a better source of valuable minerals such as calcium and zinc, and combining it with pumpkin seeds makes this dish even richer in vegetarian protein.

Serves 4

1 tbsp mild or medium (not extra virgin) olive oil, virgin rapeseed oil or coconut oil

1 red onion, finely diced

1 red pepper, deseeded and finely diced

175g (6oz) quinoa, rinsed and drained

450ml (16fl oz) hot vegetable stock

40g (1½oz) pumpkin seeds

good handful finely chopped flat-leaf parsley

good handful finely chopped baby spinach

squeeze of lemon juice

freshly ground black pepper

sea or rock salt

1 Heat the oil in a large pan or frying pan with a lid, add the onion and pepper and sauté for 10 minutes to soften.

2 Add the quinoa and stock, bring to the boil, then reduce to a simmer. Cover and cook for 15 minutes or until the quinoa has absorbed the water and softened.

3 Stir in the pumpkin seeds, parsley and spinach, then season to taste and add a squeeze of lemon juice.

Cook's Notes

Allergy suitability: gluten/wheat/dairy/yeast free (depending on stock used)

V • Can be made in advance

Health scores per serving: GL 5 • Ω • B B B

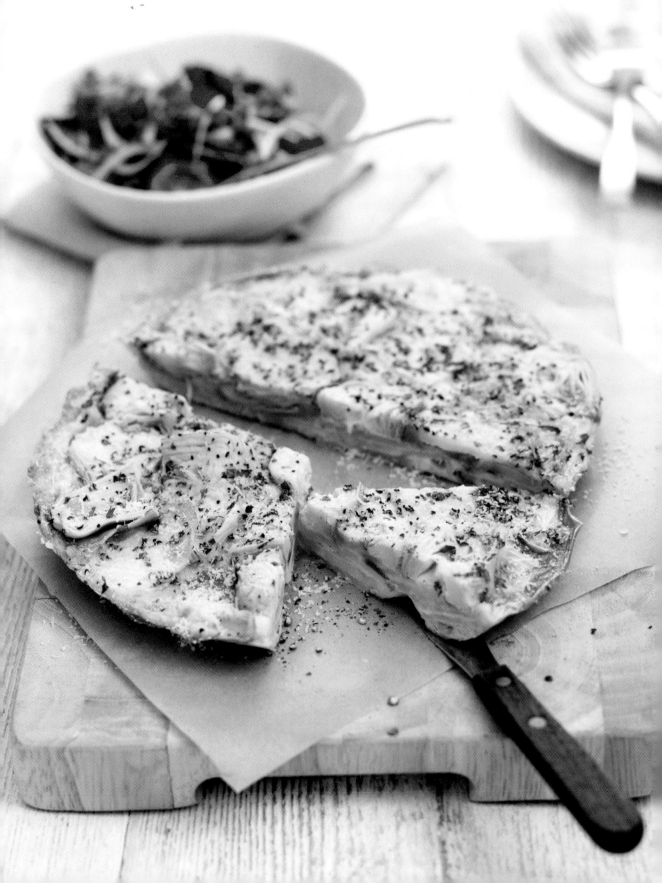

CELERIAC AND ARTICHOKE FRITTATA

A low-GL twist on a Spanish omelette, in this recipe the potato is replaced with celeriac, which is much lower in starch. Artichoke hearts are also thought to be very good for supporting the liver. Omit the Parmesan if you wish to make this dairy-free.

Serves 2

200g (7oz) celeriac, thinly sliced

2 tbsp mild or medium (not extra virgin) olive oil, virgin rapeseed oil or coconut oil

6 organic or free-range eggs

4 canned artichoke hearts, sliced

10g (¼oz) freshly grated Parmesan (optional)

freshly ground black pepper

good pinch sea or rock salt

1 tbsp finely chopped flat-leaf parsley leaves

1 Boil the celeriac slices in salted water for 12 minutes, or until tender. Drain.

2 Heat the oil in a small frying pan (one that can go under the grill) over a medium heat, add the celeriac and fry for 8 minutes or until it starts to crisp and colour.

3 Beat the eggs with the artichoke hearts, half the Parmesan and the seasoning. Preheat the grill.

4 Lower the heat under the frying pan and tip in the egg mixture. Stir quickly, then cook for 6–7 minutes, or until almost set.

4 Put the pan under the grill for 2–3 minutes, or until the top is fully cooked and golden.

5 Slide the frittata out of the pan and onto a plate or chopping board. Sprinkle with the remaining Parmesan and the parsley, slice into wedges and serve, or cool and chill, and serve cold.

Cook's Notes

Allergy suitability: gluten/wheat/dairy free (if omitting Parmesan) • V • Can be made in advance
Health scores per serving: GL 4 • BBB

SUN-DRIED TOMATO PESTO WITH CANNELLINI BEANS

This easy and delicious pesto is great stirred through pasta, quinoa or, as in this recipe, mixed with beans. It can also be dolloped onto a baked sweet potato with salad – or simply spread on bread. The recipe contains no cheese, but is an absolutely delicious pesto. It does pack a flavour punch, so if you prefer a little less garlic, by all means use fewer cloves. The pesto keeps for ten days in an airtight container in the fridge.

Makes about 10 tbsp

50g (2oz) toasted pine nuts
20 large sun-dried tomatoes
4 tbsp cider vinegar
1 tbsp Dijon mustard
6 garlic cloves, crushed

freshly ground black pepper
a little sea or rock salt
300ml (10fl oz/½ pint) extra virgin olive or rapeseed oil, or ideally a blend of both
400g can cannellini beans, rinsed and drained

1 Lightly toast the pine nuts in a dry frying pan until golden – watch carefully to stop them scorching.

2 Put the tomatoes, vinegar, mustard, garlic, pepper and salt in a food processor with the pine nuts and blend to a paste.

3 Pour in the oil and slowly blend until fairly smooth. Taste and adjust the seasoning if necessary.

4 Stir about a quarter (about 6 tbsp, or to taste) of the pesto into the beans and crush with a potato masher or lightly blitz in the food processor. Keep the remaining pesto in an airtight container in the fridge for easy meals.

Cook's Notes

Allergy suitability: gluten/wheat/dairy free • V • Can be made in advance • Suitable for freezing
Health scores per serving: GL 2 • B B B

VEGETABLE QUINOA CURRY

This dish gives you almost every colour of vegetable, making it an excellent source of antioxidants. Using quinoa instead of rice keeps the GL low and the protein content high – you won't need to serve it with rice, perhaps just with some finely diced red onion, tomato and cucumber, if you like, or on its own. The ingredients are simmered in milk but non-dairy milk works as well.

Serves 4

2 tbsp Madras curry paste

1 red onion, finely diced

1 large carrot, finely diced

½ small cauliflower, trimmed and cut into fairly small florets

175g (6oz) quinoa, rinsed and drained

4 tbsp pumpkin seeds

1 litre (1¾ pints) milk or non-dairy milk

3 tsp vegetable bouillon powder, or to taste

200g (7oz) Tenderstem broccoli (or ordinary broccoli), cut into bite-sized pieces

freshly ground black pepper

1 Heat the curry paste in a large frying pan or pan and add the onion and carrot. Fry for 5 minutes, then add the cauliflower and stir to coat.

2 Add the quinoa, pumpkin seeds, milk and bouillon powder. Stir well, then bring to the boil. Reduce the heat to a simmer, leave uncovered and cook for about 20 minutes, adding the broccoli about 5 minutes before the end of cooking to help it retain its colour and crunch.

3 Once the vegetables are al dente, the quinoa soft and most of the liquid absorbed, it is ready to serve. Taste and season accordingly.

Cook's Notes

Allergy suitability: gluten/wheat/dairy/yeast free (depending on curry paste and bouillon)

Can be made in advance

Health scores per serving: GL 9 • 🥕🥕 • Ω • Ⓑ Ⓑ Ⓑ

BAKED SWEET POTATO TOPPED WITH GOAT'S CHEESE AND SUN-DRIED TOMATOES

Sweet potatoes are thought to actively help the body to regulate blood sugar levels, making them a better choice for dieters than a standard baked potato. This delicious dish is incredibly quick and easy, and makes a lovely lunch or supper for friends, served with wilted spinach tossed in a little butter, and perhaps the Peruvian Quinoa Salad on page 116.

Serves 2

1 medium sweet potato, cut in half lengthways
a little rapeseed oil or olive oil, to coat the
    sweet potato

175g (6oz) firm goat's cheese log, sliced into
    rounds about 1cm (½in) thick
8 pieces sun-dried tomato in oil, drained

1 Preheat the oven to 190°C/375°F/Gas 5.

2 Rub the sweet potato halves with a little oil to coat, then put them cut side down, on a baking sheet and bake for 30 minutes or until soft when pierced.

3 Turn the oven off and preheat the grill until medium hot.

4 Turn each sweet potato half over and lay the cheese and tomatoes on top, alternating between the two, to cover the whole of the top of the sweet potato.

5 Pop the baking sheet under the grill and cook for a further 10 minutes or so, or until the cheese is melting and bubbling, taking care not to let the tomatoes burn (drizzling with a little oil if they are a bit dry will help prevent this).

Cook's Notes

Allergy suitability: gluten/wheat free (depending on marinade oil used for tomatoes)
Can be made in advance • V
Health scores per serving: GL 7 • 🥕 • B B

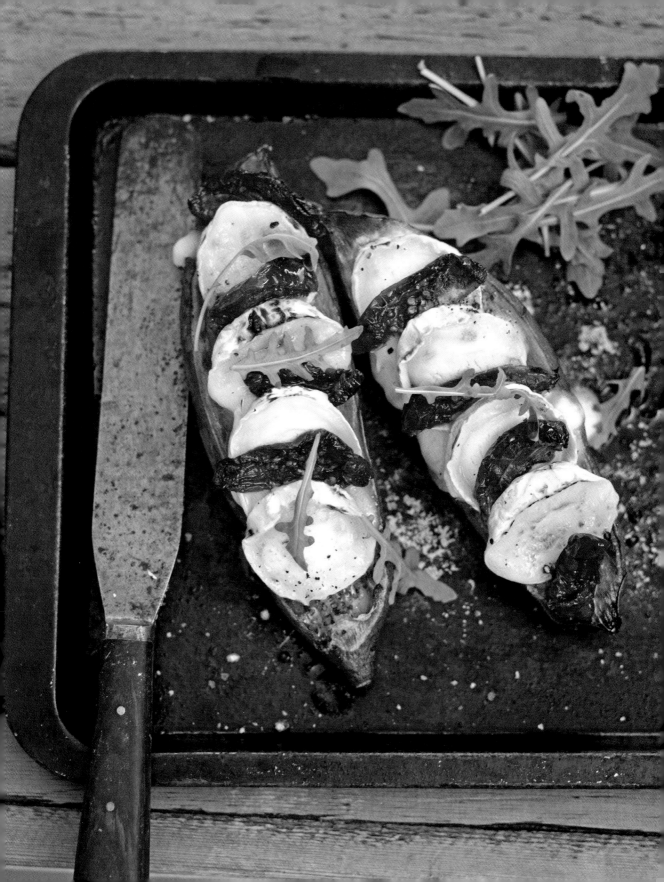

PEPPERS STUFFED WITH WILD RICE

I love wild rice, but it can take an age to cook. I recently discovered a quick-cooking version which is ready in 25 minutes but is still 100 per cent natural wild rice, with all of its high-protein, high-mineral content. Keep any excess that doesn't fit inside the pepper and serve it with salad on the side.

Serves 2

150g (5½oz) cooked wild rice (75g/3oz dried weight)

2 tbsp pumpkin seeds

4 sun-dried tomato halves, finely chopped

1 tbsp avocado oil, or extra virgin olive or virgin rapeseed oil

½ tbsp balsamic vinegar (or use lemon juice to make this yeast-free)

1 small garlic clove, crushed

1 tsp dried oregano

1 tsp finely chopped fresh basil leaves

freshly ground black pepper

a little sea or rock salt, to taste

2 red peppers

a little olive or rapeseed oil

1 Cook the rice according to the pack instructions. Preheat the oven to 200°C/400°F/Gas 6. Stir the pumpkin seeds through the rice.

2 Stir all of the remaining ingredients except the peppers and a little oil into the mixture and taste to check the seasoning.

3 Cut the tops off 2 red peppers and reserve. Slice a very thin slice from the base of each pepper to help it to stand up straight in the oven. Remove the inner pith and seeds.

4 Stuff the rice mixture into the peppers, press the mixture down firmly into the pepper, then put each one on a baking sheet and top with the reserved pepper tops. Rub a little oil into the pepper skins to prevent them from scorching. Bake for 30 minutes.

Cook's Notes

Allergy suitability: gluten/wheat/dairy/yeast free (if using lemon instead of vinegar)

Can be made in advance and chilled before cooking • V

Health scores per serving: GL 9 • 🥕🥕 • Ω • ⒷⒷ

CAULIFLOWER, CHICKPEA AND EGG CURRY

I saw this curry cooked with potatoes instead of chickpeas and it was quite delicious, so here I have devised a lower GL version, which also benefits from the chickpeas' high B vitamin content to help with methylation. Hard-boil the eggs before you start cooking, to make this simpler. Serve with brown rice or quinoa – this would take you over your 10GL limit for dieters, but is fine for weight maintenance.

Serves 4

3 tbsp coconut oil or virgin rapeseed oil

1 red, onion, diced

1 garlic clove, crushed

a thumb-sized piece of fresh root ginger, grated

2 tbsp curry paste

1 medium cauliflower, broken into florets

400g can chickpeas, rinsed and drained

400ml can full-fat coconut milk

4 hard-boiled eggs, peeled and halved lengthways

2 tbsp toasted flaked almonds (optional)

a good handful of roughly chopped fresh coriander

sea or rock salt

1 Heat a wok over a low heat, add the oil, swirl to coat, then stir in the onion and stir-fry for about 4 minutes to soften.

2 Stir the garlic and ginger into the onion mixture and cook for 1 minute.

3 Stir in the curry paste and cook for a further 1 minute before adding the cauliflower. Stir-fry to coat.

4 Add the chickpeas to the pan, then pour in the coconut milk. Stir and bring to the boil, then reduce the heat, cover the pan and simmer, stirring often, for 20–25 minutes, or until the sauce is thick and the cauliflower tender. Season to taste.

5 Put the eggs in the curry, half burying them, yolk side up, and warm through for 1–2 minutes. Sprinkle toasted flaked almonds, if using, and coriander over the top.

Cook's Notes

Allergy suitability: gluten/wheat/dairy/yeast free (depending on curry paste) • V

Can be made in advance

Health scores per serving: GL 9 • 🥕🥕🥕 • BBB

TOFU NOODLE STIR-FRY

I am not normally a big fan of tofu, but here it is packed with flavour from the ginger, garlic, soy and sesame. These ingredients also have plenty of antioxidants. If you can't find glass noodles, try soba (buckwheat) noodles, which are also, despite their name, wheat-free.

Serves 2

400g (14oz) firm tofu, patted dry with kitchen paper and cut into bite-sized cubes

4 tbsp coconut oil or virgin rapeseed oil

1cm (½in) chunk fresh root ginger, very finely chopped

1 medium red onion, sliced

1 carrot, finely sliced

150g (5½oz) sugar snap peas

150g (5½oz) glass noodles, cooked according to the pack instructions

150g (5½oz) beansprouts, rinsed

2 tbsp tamari or soy sauce

2 tbsp rice vinegar

200ml (7fl oz) vegetable bouillon or stock

juice of 1 lime

2 tbsp sesame seeds, lightly toasted

For the marinade

1 tbsp toasted sesame oil

2.5cm (1in) piece fresh root ginger, finely diced

2 garlic cloves, crushed

2 tbsp tamari or soy sauce

2 tsp rice wine vinegar

1 tsp chilli-infused oil

1 To make the marinade, mix together all the ingredients in a bowl. Stir in the tofu to coat thoroughly, then put in the fridge for at least 1 hour and preferably 3 hours or more.

2 Drain the tofu when ready to use, reserving the drained marinade for later. Heat 2 tbsp oil in a wok, add the tofu and stir-fry for 3 minutes, stirring gently as the tofu will be very soft. Remove from the wok and set to one side on a plate.

3 Heat another 2 tbsp oil in the wok, add the ginger and onion and stir-fry for 1 minute. Add the carrot and stir-fry for another 2 minutes, then add the sugar snap peas. Stir-fry for a further 5 minutes before adding the cooked noodles and beansprouts to the wok. Stir-fry to reheat and combine.

4 Pour in the tamari or soy sauce, rice vinegar, stock and remaining marinade, stir and simmer for 1 minute.

5 Ladle the stir-fry into two bowls and squeeze a little lime juice over. Sprinkle the sesame seeds on top of each portion before serving.

Cook's Notes

Allergy suitability: gluten/wheat/dairy free (depending on noodles, soy and stock) • V

Health scores per serving: GL 15 (using soba noodles, no data for glass noodles) • Ω • $\boxed{B}\,\boxed{B}\,\boxed{B}$

ACCOMPANIMENTS

THIS SECTION CONTAINS STAPLE RECIPES to help pad out your meals, from homemade breads like the Chia Loaf on page 168 to vegetable accompaniments like the Celeriac and Potato Rösti on page 172. I have focused on some more unusual options, to enliven your menus and keep boredom at bay, but you can, of course, also serve plain starch accompaniments such as brown rice, quinoa, baby new potatoes (which have the lowest GL for potatoes), lentils or wholemeal pasta (spelt is particularly good), keeping within the GL guidelines for weight loss or weight maintenance set out on page 27. Whatever you do, try to follow what nutritionists call 'the Rainbow Rule', whereby you make sure that over the course of a day or week, whichever works for you, you have managed to consume a full spectrum of different coloured fruits and vegetables. The brighter the colour, the better, as this means that the plant is particularly rich in the antioxidants that confer health benefits to you.

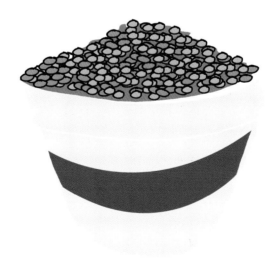

CHIA LOAF

Here I have replaced some of the flour content with ground chia seeds, to make this bread very high in nutrients. If you cannot find chia, linseeds could be used instead, although the flavour would not be as good. The loaf keeps for about five days.

Makes about 10 slices

150g (5½oz) plain wholemeal flour

1 tsp bicarbonate of soda

1 tsp salt

75g (3oz) ground chia seeds (see Resources), or use ground flax seeds

150ml (5fl oz/¼ pint) mild or medium (not extra virgin) olive oil or virgin rapeseed oil

200ml (7fl oz/⅓ pint) milk or non-dairy milk

2 free-range or organic eggs, lightly beaten

good handful of pumpkin seeds to sprinkle

1 Line a loaf tin, about 22 x 12 x 6cm (8½ x 4½ x 2.5in) with baking parchment. Preheat the oven to 150°C/300°F/Gas 2.

2 Sift the flour, bicarbonate of soda and salt into a mixing bowl (tip any leftover grains from the flour back into the mixture). Stir in the chia seeds, then add the remaining ingredients and stir well until it is all mixed together.

3 Spoon the mixture into the prepared tin and smooth it over. Sprinkle the seeds evenly over the top.

4 Bake in the centre of the oven for about 1½ hours, or until the top feels fairly hard and the mixture doesn't wobble when the tin is shaken. Leave to cool on a wire rack before storing in an airtight container.

Cook's Notes

Allergy suitability: dairy/yeast free (if using non-dairy milk) • V

Can be made in advance • Suitable for freezing

Health scores per serving (slice): GL 7 • 🥕 • Ω • Ⓑ Ⓑ Ⓑ

HERBY PUY LENTILS

This makes a great accompaniment to the Monkfish Wrapped in Parma Ham on page 148, perhaps with Peperonata (page 173), or as a complete vegetarian meal in its own right, with plenty of protein from the lentils and pumpkin seeds.

Serves 4

150g (5½oz) dried Puy lentils, rinsed and drained

1 tsp vegetable bouillon powder

3 tbsp pumpkin seeds

2 tbsp mild or medium olive oil, or virgin rapeseed oil

1 garlic clove, crushed

1 large onion, chopped

2 celery sticks, finely diced

1 tsp Italian mixed herbs

1 tsp dried oregano

1 tbsp finely chopped parsley

1 tbsp finely chopped baby spinach

2 tsp balsamic vinegar, or to taste (omit if avoiding yeast)

freshly ground black pepper

a little sea or rock salt

1 Put the lentils in a pan with the bouillon powder. Cover with cold water and bring to the boil. Reduce the heat to a simmer, then cover and cook for about 20 minutes, or until just soft to the bite. Add the pumpkin seeds halfway through cooking, to allow them to soften. Drain off any excess water from the lentils.

2 While the lentils are cooking, heat the oil in a frying pan, then add the garlic, onion and celery. Sauté gently while the lentils cook, for about 15 minutes.

3 Add the herbs and spinach to the frying pan. Turn off the heat and stir into the cooked lentils. Add the vinegar and season to taste.

Cook's Notes

Allergy suitability: gluten/wheat/dairy/yeast free (depending on bouillon and vinegar)

V • Can be made in advance

Health scores per serving: GL 7 • 🥕 • Ω • BBB

SEEDED SPELT BREAD

This mixed seed loaf first appeared in *The Perfect Pregnancy Cookbook* and is a really useful recipe to have up your sleeve. It requires no kneading or yeast to rise and it is an easy way to eat plenty of whole grains and seeds.

Serves 8–12 (freezes well)

200g (7oz) spelt flour (see Cook's Notes)

115g (4oz) mixture of raw seeds such as pumpkin, sunflower, sesame, linseed, hemp and poppy seeds, roughly ground or chopped

1 tsp sea salt

4 tsp baking powder

225ml (8fl oz) semi-skimmed milk or unsweetened non-dairy milk, such as oat or rice milk

3 medium free-range or organic eggs

5 tbsp mild or medium (not extra virgin) olive oil

50g (2oz) pumpkin seeds or other seeds, to sprinkle on top

1 Preheat the oven to 200°C/400°F/Gas 6. Line a baking tray (about 20 x 30cm/8 x 12in) with baking parchment.

2 Put the spelt flour, seeds and salt in a mixing bowl and scatter the baking powder on top. Stir to mix thoroughly.

3 Stir the milk, eggs and oil together in a bowl or jug and pour into the dry ingredients, stirring to form a loose dough. Pour into the prepared baking tray, scatter the pumpkin seeds evenly over the top and bake for 25 minutes or until golden on top and firm to the touch. Cool on a wire rack, then cut into squares and store in an airtight container.

Cook's Notes

You will find spelt flour in health-food stores.

Allergy suitability: dairy/yeast free (if using non-dairy milk) • V

Can be made in advance • Suitable for freezing

Health scores per serving (slice): GL 5 • Ω • $\boxed{B}\boxed{B}\boxed{B}$

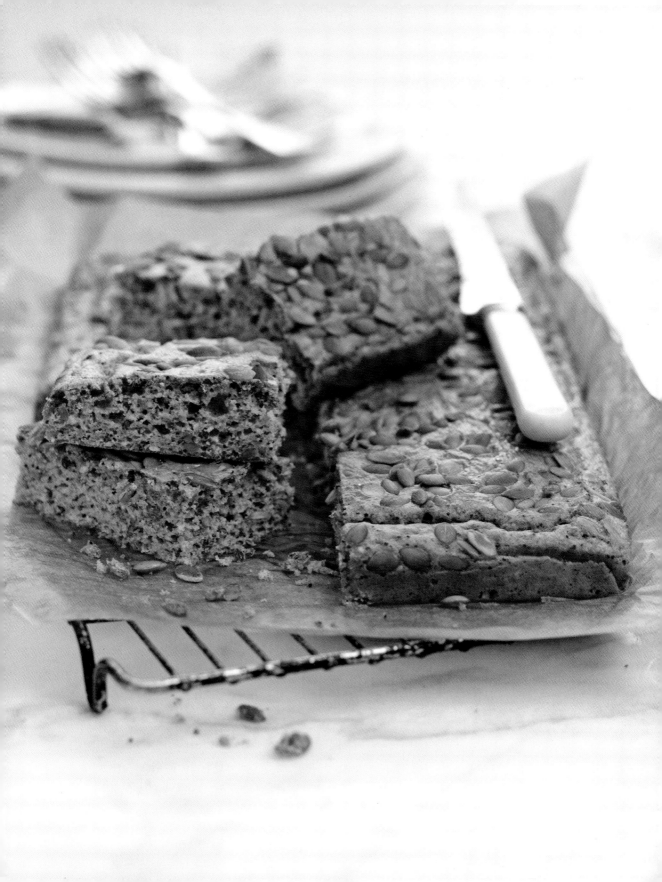

CELERIAC AND POTATO RÖSTI

Using celeriac to replace some of the potato in this rösti recipe reduces the starch to give it a lower GL. Leaving the skins on the potatoes also adds fibre to lower the GL further. This is a very nice accompaniment to a roast or served with the Venison and Chocolate Stew on page 132.

Serves 2

½ celeriac, peeled

4 small, waxy potatoes, such as Maris Pier, unpeeled (see Cook's Notes)

ground sea or rock salt

freshly ground black pepper

fresh thyme, finely chopped

1 tbsp goose fat, or butter or rapeseed oil

1 Either grate or use a mandolin to produce fine matchsticks of the celeriac and potatoes.

2 Add salt and pepper to the mixture and leave for 5–10 minutes in a sieve to allow the moisture to drain.

3 Put the mixture into a clean dish towel or muslin. Wrap and twist to wring out as much liquid as possible. Return to the fridge for 5 minutes, then repeat the process. Mix in the thyme.

4 Heat the fat or oil in a frying pan and add the mixture, either as one large cake or use rings to make smaller cakes. Aim for a thickness of 1 x 2.5cm (½ x 1in). Fry over medium heat to brown, then reduce to a low heat and cook for about 8 minutes each side, or until the mixture is cooked through.

Cook's Notes

Maris Pier potatoes are preferable to the more floury Maris Piper.

Allergy suitability: gluten/wheat/dairy/yeast free • Can be made in advance • V

Health scores per serving: GL 7 • B B

PEPERONATA

Soft, sweet and sticky Mediterranean flavours, delicious served warm or cold with meat, fish, cheese or quinoa. Try it with the Celeriac and Artichoke Frittata on page 159. The bright colours demonstrate the dish's high antioxidant content. You can add a glug of red wine or balsamic vinegar to the mixture while cooking, if you wish.

Serves 6

8 tbsp olive oil (see Cook's Notes)

9 garlic cloves, sliced

3 red onions, cut into wedges

6 red, yellow and/or orange peppers, thinly sliced lengthways

350g (12oz) cherry tomatoes

150g (5½oz) good olives, such as Kalamata

2 tsp dried oregano or 1 tbsp chopped fresh oregano

freshly ground black pepper

freshly torn basil leaves, to garnish

1 Heat the oil in a large pan (as large as you have), add the garlic and onions and gently sauté for about 10 minutes to soften.

2 Add the peppers, cover and cook for a further 10 minutes before adding the tomatoes, olives and oregano.

3 Simmer, covered, for a further 45 minutes or until the tomatoes have burst and produced a wonderfully sticky, gloopy sauce amid the soft vegetables. Season and scatter with basil. Serve warm or at room temperature.

Cook's Notes

I like to use half medium/mild oil and the other half extra virgin, for the best flavour.

Allergy suitability: gluten/wheat/dairy/yeast free (depending if the olives are stored in vinegar or not)

V • Can be made in advance • Suitable for freezing

Health scores per serving: GL 1 • 🥕🥕🥕🥕🥕 • Ⓑ Ⓑ Ⓑ

STIR-FRIED CHOI SUM IN OYSTER SAUCE

Choi sum is a typically Chinese stir-fry vegetable, which has a wonderful flavour and texture. It can be found in Chinese supermarkets, but use pak choi if you can't get hold of it. The addition of plenty of ginger helps to make this dish strongly anti-inflammatory.

Serves 2

1½ tbsp mild oil such as rapeseed
  or coconut oil
5cm (2in) piece fresh ginger root, shredded or
  very finely slivered

large bunch choi sum, split into stems and
  leaves
3 tbsp oyster sauce

1 Heat the oil in a wok. Add the ginger and stir-fry for 1 minute.

2 Add the choi sum stems and cook for 2 minutes.

3 Add the choi sum leaves and cook for a further 3 minutes.

4 Reduce the heat and add the oyster sauce. Serve immediately.

Cook's Notes
Allergy suitability: gluten/wheat/dairy free (depending on the oyster sauce) • V
Health scores per serving: GL 1 • 🥕🥕 • Ⓑ

SAVOY CABBAGE WITH CHESTNUTS

This delicious accompaniment contains lots of B vitamins and has a suitable low-GL carbohydrate content, as chestnuts are a good source of slow-releasing energy. As with the Braised Kale with Almonds on page 176, adding nuts helps to enliven green vegetable dishes.

Serves 2–4

1 tbsp goose fat, coconut oil or mild or medium (not extra virgin) olive oil, or virgin rapeseed oil

1 medium savoy cabbage, outer leaves and tough core removed, then finely shredded

200g vacuum pack peeled, cooked chestnuts, broken into pieces

1 tbsp hot vegetable stock

ground white pepper

1 Heat the fat or oil in a large frying pan. Add the cabbage and stir-fry for 1–2 minutes, then add the chestnuts.

2 Add the stock, stir and cover. Cook for 3–5 minutes or until the cabbage has softened.

3 Season with a sprinkle of pepper – you may not need salt.

Cook's Notes

Allergy suitability: gluten/wheat/dairy/yeast free (depending on stock used)

V (if using oil rather than goose fat) • Can be made in advance

Health scores per serving (when serving 4): GL 1 • B B

BRAISED KALE WITH ALMONDS

Kale never sounds desperately exciting, but this dish has converted me completely. Braising it in bouillon makes it wonderfully soft and well flavoured, with the almonds providing a little crunch. Kale is, of course, a cruciferous vegetable and its dark green colour shows how rich it is in antioxidants.

Serves 2

50g (2oz) flaked almonds

1 tbsp butter or dairy-free spread suitable for cooking, or coconut oil (see Cook's Notes)

1 garlic clove, crushed

115g (4oz) curly kale, stems removed, sliced

4 tbsp hot vegetable bouillon

freshly ground black pepper

1 Toast the almonds in a dry frying pan over a low heat for a few minutes or until lightly browned, taking care not to let them burn.

2 Add the butter, spread or oil and swirl it about the pan to coat (take the pan off the heat temporarily to stop it burning), then throw in the garlic and stir.

3 Add the kale and bouillon to the pan, stir, then cover and allow to steam-fry for about 2 minutes or until the kale is tender. If the pan runs dry, throw in a little more stock or water. Season with black pepper, then serve.

Cook's Notes

Butter gives the best flavour to this dish by far.

Allergy suitability: gluten/wheat/dairy/yeast free (depending on butter and bouillon)

V • Can be made in advance

Health scores per serving: GL 1 • 🥕 • BB

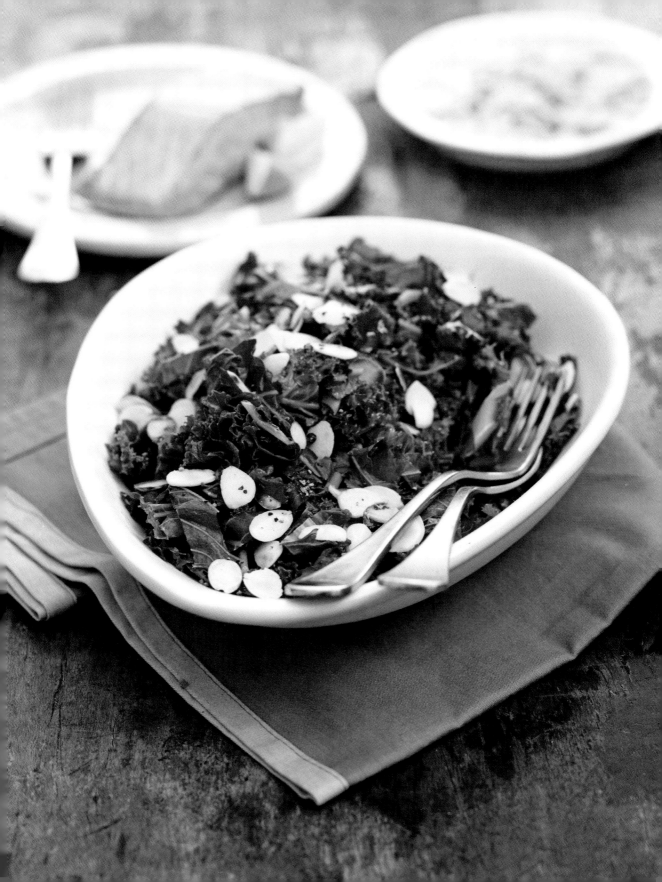

PUDDINGS AND SWEET TREATS

IF, LIKE ME, YOU HAVE A SWEET TOOTH, you'll be reassured to hear that I have made sure that there are plenty of options to give yourself a treat, without derailing all your efforts to be healthy. In these recipes I have focused on antioxidant-rich fruits, such as berries and pomegranate, to boost your daily ORAC intake as well as providing natural sweetness. I have steered clear of grains in all but one recipe, where I use whole-grain rough oatcakes (the Chocolate Crunchies shown below), in order to focus on lower carbohydrate ingredients such as eggs, yogurt and fruit. I use xylitol (see page 67) as a sweetener in preference to sugar as it has a very low GL and is also suitable for diabetics. It can be used in a 1:1 substitution for ordinary sugar. Lastly, you might be surprised to see chocolate featuring in two recipes, but in fact good-quality chocolate with a high cocoa solid content of anything above 70 per cent will not only taste delicious but it will also contain valuable iron and antioxidants, not to mention tryptophan, which plays a part in controlling sleep and mood.

All in all, these recipes are intended to provide something to look forward to at the end of a meal, without deviating from the recommendations in Part One.

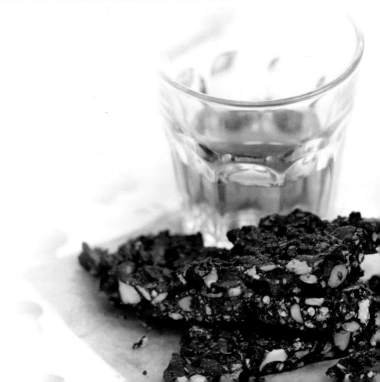

CHOCOLATE CRUNCHIES

This is a really useful recipe; make a batch, cut it up and keep it in the freezer. It can be served from frozen, which makes it wonderfully chewy and a little like a chocolate ice cream bar, and is a brilliant standby for when you have unexpected guests. It may taste decadent, but the ingredients are all very nutritious, the dark chocolate included.

Serves 10

200g (7oz) dark chocolate, 70% cocoa solids, broken into chunks
125g (4½oz) rough oatcakes
50g (2oz) goji berries
50g (2oz) Brazil nuts, roughly chopped
50g (2oz) pumpkin seeds
4 tsp ground mixed spice
2 tsp ground cinnamon
50g (2oz) hazelnut butter or unsalted peanut butter (see Cook's Notes)

1 Melt the chocolate, stirring occasionally, in a heatproof bowl over a pan of gently simmering water, making sure the base of the bowl doesn't touch the water.

2 Put the oatcakes into a mixing bowl and crumble into small pieces. Stir in the goji berries, nuts, seeds and spices.

3 Stir the nut butter into the melted chocolate and mix until fairly smooth. Stir the chocolate mixture into the remaining ingredients, making sure the ingredients are evenly coated.

4 Spread the mixture over a baking sheet and put in the fridge or freezer to chill and harden. Break into shards or cut into rough pieces when set, ready to serve.

Cook's Notes

You can also use tahini instead of hazelnut butter, but you may need to sweeten the mixture further with a little xylitol or honey, as it is rather bitter.
Allergy suitability: wheat/dairy/yeast free (depending on oatcakes) • V
Can be made in advance; keeps indefinitely in the freezer • Suitable for freezing
Health scores per serving: GL 8 • 🥕🥕🥕🥕 • Ω • B̄B̄

COCONUT CUPS

This recipe is not dissimilar to a coconut brûlée, albeit minus the delicious burnt sugar topping. Using coconut milk for a jelly makes this rich in medium-chain triglycerides or MCTs, which are good fats that the body tends to use as fuel rather than storing as fat.

Serves 4 (larger coffee cups) or 8 (espresso cups)

4 leaf gelatine sheets

400ml can full-fat coconut milk

3 tbsp xylitol (or caster sugar)

2 tbsp desiccated coconut

1 Soak the gelatine in a little cold water for 5 minutes or until softened.

2 Meanwhile, put the coconut milk and xylitol or sugar into a pan and simmer to allow the crystals to dissolve.

3 Take the gelatine leaves out the water and squeeze to remove as much water as possible, then add to the coconut milk and stir to dissolve completely.

4 Put four coffee cups or eight espresso cups on a tray, then carefully pour the liquid into each, to avoid splashing. Put the tray in the fridge for at least 4 hours, or overnight, to allow the jelly to set.

5 Toast the desiccated coconut in a dry frying pan until golden, then allow to cool, and sprinkle over the top of each jelly before serving.

Cook's Notes

Allergy suitability: gluten/wheat/dairy/yeast free

Health scores per serving (espresso cups): GL 2

CHOCOLATE ESPRESSO MOUSSE

Dark chocolate is rich in antioxidants and iron. The raw egg yolk in this mousse also provides plenty of methylation-boosting nutrients. Espresso coffee contains less caffeine than filter coffee and also has a high ORAC score. Use decaf coffee if you prefer, or make a Chocolate Orange Mousse by replacing the espresso with freshly squeezed orange juice.

Serves 4–6

200g (7oz) dark chocolate, 70% cocoa solids, broken into chunks

6 medium organic or free-range eggs, separated
4 tbsp espresso coffee

1 Melt the chocolate, stirring occasionally, in a heatproof bowl over a pan of gently simmering water, making sure the base of the bowl doesn't touch the water. Set it to one side to cool for a few minutes, so that it does not cook the egg when you mix the two together.

2 Beat the egg yolks with the coffee, then stir into the melted chocolate.

3 Put the egg whites into a clean, grease-free bowl and whisk until they form stiff peaks. Add a large spoonful to the chocolate mixture, mixing well to loosen the consistency. Gently fold in the remaining egg white, then spoon into a serving bowl, cover and chill for 2 hours or until set, preferably overnight.

Cook's Notes

Allergy suitability: gluten/wheat/dairy/yeast free • V • Can be made in advance
Health scores per serving (for 6 servings): GL 4 • 🥕🥕🥕🥕🥕 • Ⓑ

PINEAPPLE, POMEGRANATE AND MINT FRUIT SALAD

If you are just eating this yourself and want to cut down on steps to save time, the pineapple and pomegranate alone makes a naturally sweet, refreshing end to a meal that aids digestion, otherwise, the mint and sweetened citrus juice adds extra flavour.

Serves 2

⅓ ripe pineapple

½ pomegranate

2 tsp xylitol (or brown sugar)

2 tbsp lime or lemon juice

½ tbsp finely chopped fresh mint leaves

1 Slice the pineapple as thinly as you possibly can, then neatly cut away the edges. Arrange the slices overlapping each other on a serving plate or individual plates.

2 Cut the pomegranate in half and remove the seeds from one half, discarding all the membranes (keep the other half in the fridge and add to fruit salads or yoghurt, or munch as a snack). Scatter the seeds over the pineapple slices.

3 Stir the xylitol or sugar into the lime or lemon juice, so that it starts to dissolve.

4 Spoon the sweetened juice over the fruit, then scatter the mint on top.

Cook's Notes

Allergy suitability: gluten/wheat/dairy/yeast free • V • Can be made up to 2–3 hours in advance and chilled until needed

Health scores per serving: GL 4 • 🥕🥕🥕🥕

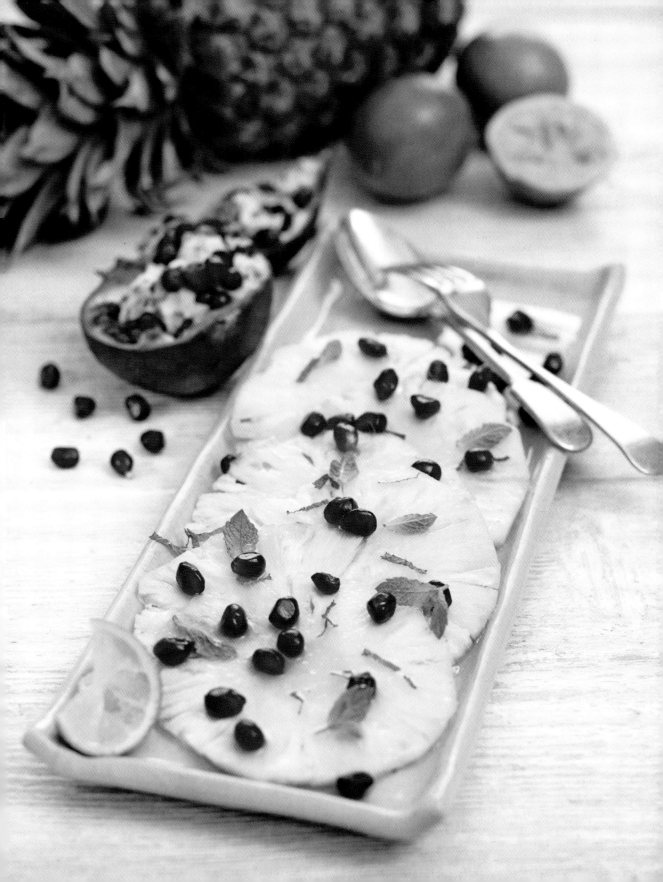

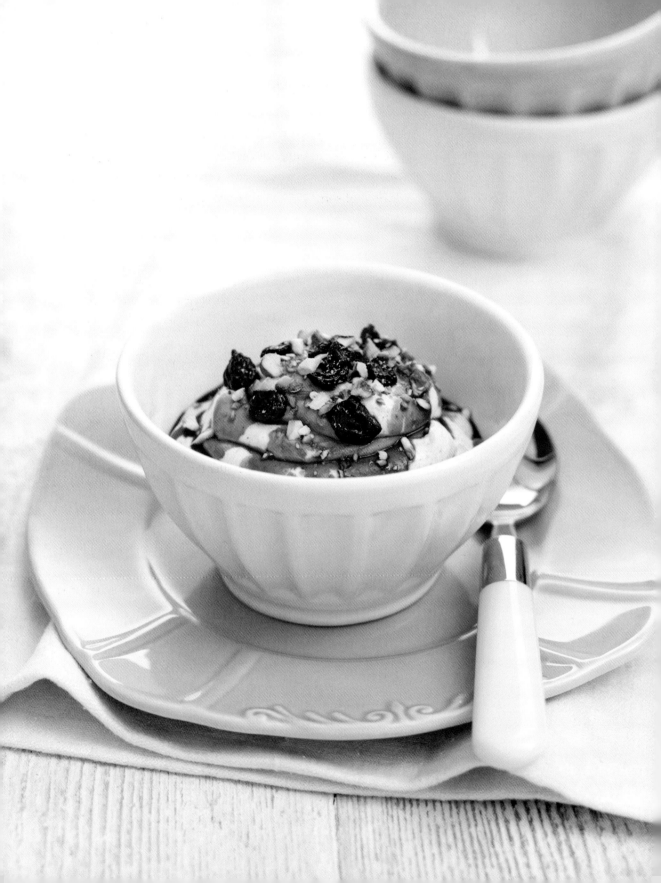

GREEK YOGHURT AND CHERRY POTS

This is a very good pudding in its own right, but take a look at the ORAC score below to see just how good it is for you too. Montmorency cherries have been shown to have particularly high antioxidant levels, and pistachio nuts are reported to have anti-inflammatory effects. The addition of some cinnamon serves to help your body keep blood sugar levels balanced.

Serves 1

½ tsp ground cinnamon

6 heaped tbsp Greek yoghurt, or use sheep's or goat's yoghurt, or even soya yoghurt

2 squirts Cherry Active concentrated Montmorency cherry juice (see Resources), or use berry juice

½ tbsp dried Montmorency cherries or use ordinary dried cherries, blueberries or cranberries, roughly chopped (see Cook's Notes)

1 tbsp unsalted, shelled pistachio nuts or walnuts, roughly chopped

1 Stir the cinnamon into the yoghurt, mixing well.

2 Spoon the yoghurt mixture into a short glass, or a pot or small bowl.

3 Pour the Cherry Active or berry juice over the yoghurt, then scatter the dried cherries or berries and nuts on top.

Cook's Notes

Montmorency cherries are available from Cherry Active (see Resources). If you use ordinary dried cherries, avoid the luridly coloured ones that you used to see on top of trifles.

Allergy suitability: gluten/wheat/yeast free • V • Can be made in advance (sits happily in the fridge for a couple of hours)

Health scores per serving: GL 7 • 🥕🥕🥕🥕🥕🥕🥕🥕 • Ω • B̄ B̄

BLUEBERRY JELLIES

This is a delicious as a guilt-free, high-ORAC pudding. You can top with a layer of Greek yoghurt or mascarpone to make this a little more decadent and delicious.

Serves 4 or 8

4 leaf gelatine sheets

375g (13oz) blueberries

300ml (10fl oz/½ pint) 100% blueberry juice (or an unsweetened blueberry or berry juice drink)

1 Soak the gelatine in a little cold water for 5 minutes or until softened.

2 Meanwhile, put 300g (11oz) of the berries and the juice into a pan, bring to the boil, then reduce the heat, cover and simmer gently for 5 minutes to allow the fruit to soften. Pour the mixture though a sieve into a large bowl, pressing firmly to squeeze as much flesh and juice out of the fruit as possible, and leaving behind the skins.

3 Take the gelatine leaves out the water and squeeze to remove as much water as possible, then add to the blueberry juice and stir to dissolve completely.

4 Divide the remaining blueberries between the bases of four ramekins, or eight espresso cups. Put all the ramekins or cups on a tray, then carefully pour the jelly liquid on top to avoid splashing. Put the tray in the fridge for at least 4 hours, or overnight, to allow the jelly to set.

Cook's Notes

Allergy suitability: gluten/wheat/dairy/yeast free

Health scores per serving (for 8 servings): GL 4 • 🥕 🥕 🥕

PINEAPPLE SORBET

Pineapple is a great choice to end a meal, as it contains bromelain, an enzyme that helps to breakdown protein to aid digestion. To check that it is ripe, try pulling one of the pineapple leaves from the top – if it comes away easily, the pineapple should be ripe. I keep pots of this sorbet in the freezer for a healthy alternative to ice cream to give to my toddler. It more than passes the children's taste test.

Serves 4
1 ripe pineapple
splash of milk or non-dairy milk

1 Remove the top and skin of the pineapple, cutting away any tough bits.

2 Roughly slice the pineapple, then put into a blender.

3 Add a splash of milk, enough to help you blend the mixture, then blitz to a smooth, slushy consistency.

4 Put in a container with a lid and freeze for a few hours until set. Remove from the freezer about 20 minutes before serving to melt slightly, in order to make it easier to serve and eat.

Cook's Notes
Allergy suitability: gluten/wheat/dairy/yeast free (depending on milk) • V

Can be made in advance • Suitable for freezing

Health scores per serving: GL 5 •

RESOURCES

Test kits

Homocysteine and food allergy tests Homocysteine and food allergy (IgG ELISA tests) are available through York Test Laboratories, using a home-test kit where you can take your own pinprick blood sample and return it to the lab for analysis. Visit www.yorktest.com, or call freephone (UK) 0800 074 6185. These test kits are also available from www.totallynourish.com.

Ingredients

Cherry Active is sold in a highly concentrated juice format. Mix a 30ml (2 tbsp) serving with 250ml (9fl oz) water to make a deliciously healthy, low-GL cherry juice. Each 946ml bottle contains the juice from over 3,000 cherries – that's half a tree's worth – and contains a month's supply. Cherry Active is also available as a dried cherry snack and in capsules. For more information and to order, visit www.totallynourish.com or call freephone (UK) 0800 085 7749.

Montmorency Cherries Although all fresh fruits, especially cherries, are full of goodness, the Montmorency cherry variety has been found to be packed with high levels of antioxidants and flavonoids, including Anthocyanin and Melotonin.
Scientific evidence suggests that these compounds may help maintain healthy joints, normal uric acid levels and healthy sleep patterns and help muscles recover quickly from sport and training.

Virgin coconut oil For superb-quality, fairly traded, certified organic virgin coconut oil (retail/wholesale) contact Coconut Connections Ltd, 5 Sycamore Dene, Chesham, Bucks HP5 3JT. Phone 01494 771419 or order from their website www.virgincoconutoil.co.uk

Chia seeds, the highest vegetarian source of omega-3, are available from Totally Nourish. www.totallynourish.com. If you'd like to find out more, here are two useful websites – www.eatchia.com and www.drcoateschia.com.

Sugar alternative – **XyloBrit (xylitol)** is a low-GL natural sugar alternative – available in health-food stores and from www.totallynourish.com or call freephone (UK) 0800 085 7749.

Cooking pans

Scanpan is one of the world's leading producers of non-stick cookware. Scanpan has also developed Green Tek, a non-stick coating that is 100 per cent free from perfluorooctanoic acid (PFOA) and perfluorooctane sulfonate (PFOS) chemicals, to protect the health of users and the environment. Together with Scanpan's patented ceramic titanium technology, Green Tek forms one of the most resistant non-stick coatings on the market. This makes Scanpan much longer lasting than conventional non-stick cookware. Visit www.scanpan.com for more information.

Green Pan does not use harmful polytetrafluoroethylene (PTFE) coatings, but instead uses Thermolon non-stick technology, which is heat-resistant up to high temperatures so that if you overheat your pan, even up to 450°C/850°F, no toxic fumes will be released and the coating will not blister or peel. This makes Green Pan much longer lasting than conventional non-stick cookware. Green Pan non-stick pots and pans are also the first to be made with a non-stick coating made of minerals instead of plastics, to limit environmental impact. Visit www.green-pan.com for more information.

Other recommendations

Nutrition Consultancy in Commercial Catering
The Russell Partnership is the UK's leading strategic catering and hospitality consultancy offering advice and assistance on the commercial application of nutrition. Services include Nutritional Audits, leading to Food for the Brain accreditation, training and workshops on the commercial application of nutrition. Visit www.russellpartnership.com or call (0) 20 7665 1888 for more details.

Yano Parents often face a particular struggle to incorporate healthy eating principles into their children's diets. The Yano website offers advice to parents from experts in the fields of children's nutrition (from author Fiona McDonald Joyce), behaviour and development, as well as providing a forum for parents to share their own experiences and support each other. For more information visit www.yano.co.uk.

Index